Arrest Ageing

For Margaret

Rachel C. Harper

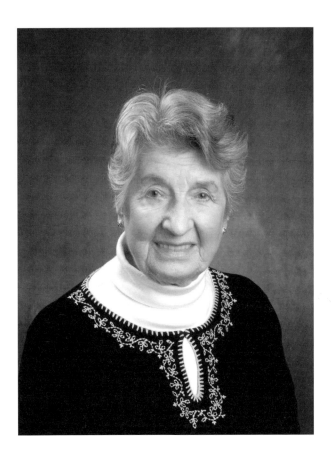

ABOUT THE AUTHOR

Rachel Campbell-Hayes is a very fit and outgoing octogenarian. She does not feel she is retired because she has remained as active and busy as when she started her working life in fashion in Glasgow aged sixteen. Progressing from fashion buyer to housekeeper, to welfare work, to floristry to founding a babywear shop aged seventy, she also coped with being a widow at age thirty-four, with a young child to bring up. The exercises included in this book were developed by the author in her sixties when she found class-work too demanding and exhausting but believed there was a way for older people to keep fit through specially designed exercises that took account of their particular needs.

Arrest Ageing

An Exercise Programme
for the Over-fifties
to Delay the Signs of
Ageing

by

Rachel Campbell Hayes

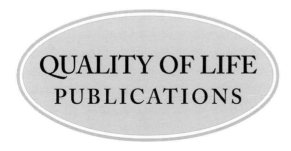

QUALITY OF LIFE
PUBLICATIONS

Copyright © Rachel Campbell Hayes 2001

First published in 2001 by Quality of Life Publications
26 Bramble Drive
Edinburgh
EH4 8BP

Distributed by Gazelle Book Services Limited
Falcon House, Queen Square
Lancaster, England LA1 1RN

British Library Cataloguing in Publication Data
A catalogue record for this book is available from the British Library

ISBN 0-9540413-0-5

Typeset by Amolibros, Watchet, Somerset
This book production has been managed by Amolibros
Printed and bound by T J International, Padstow, Cornwall, England

Contents

Introduction

Welcome to my programme of exercises, designed to help you revitalise and get the most out of your life.

I have compiled this programme of breathing and physical exercises, suitable for both men and women of a mature age. You would probably like to know what prompted me to do this, at a time when there are already many aids to keeping fit – videos demonstrating exercise programmes, exercise programmes on television, and a great many books of course. Excellent though all that material is, I have so far not been able to find something that, in every respect, really suits me.

We do not always have classes that are both easily available in terms of location and time of day, and that have appropriate exercises for mature people. Most books, videos and television programmes, interesting and well presented as most of them are, are mainly targeted at a younger age group.

This programme is meant for people of fifty years of age and beyond. It is hoped that you find it so beneficial that you will want to incorporate it into your lifestyle on a permanent basis. It will serve as a great invigorator in revitalising you, and will make you feel you have more energy and are able to enjoy life more. From my experience, this programme can serve you well into your eighties. It may well be practical to continue it into your nineties, though that I cannot yet write about, as I have not yet tried it!

I can see no reason why I won't be able to continue with the programme for many years to come. I endeavour to present an honest view of it – one that is tried and tested – and one that doesn't come with claims I cannot justify. To ensure the validity of the principles on which the programme is based, and the safety of the exercises themselves, I enlisted the help of two friends who have had formal training and many years' experience in physical education, exercise programming and sports coaching. They have also been responsible for programmes of classes targeted at the older age groups, and so have experience of the problems and benefits of such programmes, as well as the features that encourage people to keep up their exercise programmes over extended periods of time.

As I write this I am in my eighty-seventh year. I have evolved this programme from my own experience of yoga and other forms of exercise (such as walking, swimming and aquafit). All these activities I took up after I was sixty, and after I had completed a very full working life – a life that left little time for sport or organised exercise for my own benefit. I do not write this as someone who has been a fitness enthusiast all my life, nor as someone who has never had aches and pains. Like many of you, I suffer from a certain amount of arthritis. I am, however, fully convinced that this programme of exercise plays a major part in keeping me very mobile and active for my age. Neither do I write this as someone who devotes most of my days to exercise. I believe your programme must be adaptable, and able to fit a busy life. There is no joy in being fit if it takes all your waking hours to achieve it, and leaves you no time to do the other things you are striving to be fit for! Furthermore I don't lead the deprived life of reduced eating and drinking in order to manage my body and keep my weight down. The social element of eating and drinking together with friends is a very important aspect of my life, therefore I enjoy a good varied diet, taking wine with my evening meal most days. Striving for a body that will enable you to have the quality of life that you want in your later years must not become a penance in itself.

It is not an overstatement to say that exercise of this nature has a rejuvenating effect. It is not competitive. It is not exhausting. It requires no further expense. I thoroughly recommend it as one of the best investments in both money and time that you have ever made. Your time and commitment are the only things you have to give for a new lease of life. A revitalised body and the capacity to get more out of your later years is a big reward for a little time and effort.

Perhaps you are either just on the verge of retirement or retired already, still working out what you are going to do with your later years. As part of that planning process you may be wondering how long you will remain active and able to get around easily. Perhaps you have been retired for a while and feel it's all very well but you lack the energy and drive to do very much with it. Perhaps you are still at work and feeling the stress of all those deadlines, juggling these and home commitments, and feeling all the tension that kind of pressure brings. In all cases I feel that a little effort put into this programme will offer great rewards, in terms of feeling so much more fit and able, so much more full of energy, and so better adapted not only to the tasks required of you, but the things you would really like to do, for your own fulfilment.

If you have not been a fitness-class enthusiast so far in your life, or if you like many have made short but unsustained efforts at exercise and fitness over the years, it is unlikely in your later years you will want to start very energetic and exhausting daily routines. This does not mean you cannot have a body to be proud of, and one that enables you to enjoy your later years to a maximum.

Are you fifty years of age or more?
Are you approaching retirement?
Do you feel tired and weary?
Do you move less easily than you used to?
Would you like to feel ten years younger?
Do you want to have an active and interesting retirement?
Do you feel good and want to stay that way?

If any of these statements applies to you then this book has material that if used will help you to feel better and get more out of your life.

I would like you to believe what you read, because taken seriously the programme can make an amazing change to your later years. This can be in relation to your general mobility and the effect that such mobility has on the ease of everyday living. It can also be in relation to your muscle tone, which has a major effect on how you look, and is related to your strength levels. It can also be in terms of your energy level and ability to do other things and get more out of life.

It is an accepted fact that we are living longer, but if we are to enjoy our later years we require a fit and active body and mind. Living for longer, which is mainly due to the decrease in infectious diseases, and the improvements in medical care, is not a great achievement in itself if we are not able to use that time to our benefit and enjoy it. *Quantity* of life alone is not enough – it is also about the *quality* of it.

The programme is for mature men and women, and is designed to meet the demands of living in a stressful society, whose lifestyles no longer provide the range of exercise opportunities that, for example, was part of everyday life for our grandparents. All our labour-saving devices in the home, our less physically demanding working lives, our ever increasing use of the motor car, combined with our television and computer controlled leisure activities, mean we are less active. We are certainly less active than our bodies require to keep in good shape. We have to make a positive decision to do something about this, particularly if we want to enjoy an active later life. The advantages that technology has brought, in reducing our everyday physical labour, together with medical advances, though having significantly increased our life expectancy, could end in conflict, if the one makes us unable to benefit from the other.

This programme is done at a pace that does not exhaust or injure you. Do keep in mind the fact that you can carry this programme on into your eighties.

The principal element of the programme is a very personal study of your body and mind, using breathing and exercising in a really slow way. Although you move slowly, you are still exercising your joints and muscles.

If you feel some of the positions in the exercises are demanding, you should recover by using slow deep breathing before continuing. The breathing is just as important as the exercises and held positions. The majority of us do not use our full lung capacity, but breathe in a very shallow way. Deep breathing improves the oxygen supply to all parts of the body. Oxygen is essential for life. If we do not have it we die, and if we do not get sufficient of it circulating round our body, we operate below our optimum. We are obviously conscious of our lack of adequate oxygen when we run for a bus or some similar very physical task, because that leaves us gasping for breath. This applies equally to those situations where we *aren't* conscious of the body's need for oxygen. Most ongoing functions, such as those of the brain, come into this category. So, I am going to ask you to establish in your mind that breathing is a very powerful tool, and central to the entire programme. Deep breathing also helps to make a tranquil mind. Many of the held positions are taken from yoga; and many are modified to enable you to perform them in later years. The range of exercises chosen is meant to benefit the entire body. It is not wise to pick out the ones you are good at and like, as this will mean you are not caring for all parts of the body, nor are you getting a well balanced workout. On the other hand, you may not always have time to complete the whole programme at once, and some suggestions on shorter balanced programmes are included in a later section. This would enable you on occasions to cover the programme in two or three phases, rather than miss out altogether. In the early stages, when you are learning the exercises, and possibly still reading some of the instructions, it will take you a bit longer to work through and complete than is the case when you know the exercises well. During the learning stage you may want to do only some of the exercises at a time, and work your way through the whole programme over two or three sessions. There are also occasions when you will not have sufficient time to do the whole programme in one go, and so will want to use the series of shortened sessions.

I would ask you to re-read this introductory section again before you start any workout, as there are important principles and ideas to absorb to help you get the maximum benefit from your participation.

Summary of important ideas

➤ The programme is designed for the over-fifties

➤ It aims to improve your mobility, muscle tone and breathing

➤ It aims to increase your level of activity and enjoyment in your later years

➤ Through enhancing your breathing you will revitalise your mind and body

Prior to starting any programme of exercise it is advisable to check with your doctor if you think there is any possibility that it might not be recommended for you.

Getting started

1.1 What to wear

Now, a few thoughts on what to wear and other steps to take before you can start in earnest. The ladies should wear really baggy shorts or stretch tights, leggings or jogging bottoms and a sweater. I personally prefer to work with my feet covered in the cold weather – this can be either with socks or soft, well fitting lightweight shoes. Men should wear baggy shorts or jogging bottoms and a T-shirt, sweatshirt or sweater. The important thing is that the clothing is comfortable, does not restrict your movement in any way, and keeps you adequately warm without getting too hot. Clothing is personal and you should be guided by what feels comfortable and allows you to move freely. It is also, to a great extent, seasonal. For example, in summer you can strip off to something very light and loose with bare feet, while in winter you will possibly need an extra layer of loose, comfortable warm clothing.

1.2 Your working space

It is important that your exercising space is adequate in size and is warm, as you will not work well if you are cold – in fact your joints and muscles will rebel! A cold body and cold conditions can lead to injury.

You will require a rug or mat to perform on. You may also require a small thin cushion under your head, as some people are not confident or at ease lying absolutely flat on the floor. If your chin always seems to be higher than your forehead when lying flat you will require a cushion to help tip your head slightly forward.

I personally like very soft music playing in the background. The choice is yours but it should be played low and should be smooth and melodic, rather than loud and strident.

1.3 Concerned about whether you will manage?

If you feel lacking in confidence over some of the postures, bear in mind that you are working on the floor. Clowns in the circus ring practise rolling about in order not to injure themselves in their performance. The rock-'n'-roll exercise that is featured near the start of the programme is excellent to give you the confidence to move around the floor without injury.

If you are not used to exercise you must start gently. If you feel awkward at the start, if you are not able to do some of the movements or positions fully, this is natural and acceptable. If you have any reservations or any significant health problems you should consult your doctor, prior to starting, to reassure yourself and enable you to participate with confidence and not anxiety. It is rare but if you feel slight nausea, dizziness or poor balance, go slowly and keep focusing on breathing in and out, and pause when you need to stabilise yourself. The condition soon passes. If your balance is really poor do not have your feet together in any of the standing warm-up exercises, and do not exercise with the eyes closed. Instead stand with the feet apart and keep the eyes open. It is helpful in all the exercises to focus your gaze, either straight forward or forward and slightly upward. This helps concentration. Many of the exercises prompt you about where your gaze should focus.

If you have a weight problem, particularly in the abdominal or hip region, it can be difficult lowering yourself to the floor and rising again. This does not mean the programme is not for you. It means that you use a simple and easy technique to help you get up and down in the early stages. Start working with a chair close beside your rug or mat. Use the chair to lean on to help you get down onto your knees, then sit over onto your hip and with the aid of your hands bring the legs forward, then stretch out to lie flat on the back, remembering that you may want a small thin cushion to put under your head. Endeavour to become used to this position before you attempt other postures. Stretch out fully, legs straight, feet turned out, hands relaxed by your side, palms up, chin down and shoulders away from ears. Just lie in this position breathing deeply. That alone is good for you as it allows you to relax and requires a minimum of effort. When you are ready to rise, go through the same procedure in reverse. Sit up by placing both hands under your waist, palms down and push slowly and vigorously into a sitting position. Bring the knees up with the feet on the floor, roll sideways onto your hip, then raise yourself to your knees, then to your feet, using your hands and the chair to support you. The secret is to take time, and with repetition it will make a difference. Each time, make a note of your progress – however slow. Remember you are not in a class with your eye on your neighbour (whom you imagine to be very much slimmer, fitter and more agile than you). This may destroy your confidence from the start.

I have to cover these points because many people starting this programme have a weight problem. I reiterate: this does not mean that the programme is not for you. It's rather the reverse. Granted you will have to work harder, but you will get results (and I know how good you will feel after just a few weeks). You do not require travelling to a class in bad weather, as you can set up your own workspace and music. There is no competition, and so your progress can never be hindered. Your home is your workspace, and your daily routine is the timetable into which you fit your exercise.

At the beginning I pointed out that the emphasis is on the slow movement and deep breathing that enables you to continue much later in life than most popular faddish methods of keeping fit. Please bear this in mind.

1.4 Think of the benefits as you go along

I am sure you are interested to know what conditions can greatly benefit from the programme. There are many that will improve if the muscles of the body are well toned and stretched. These include backache, arthritis, headaches and cramp. Other conditions, such as asthma and insomnia, benefit from the breathing exercises. Yet others such as stress, indigestion, poor circulation, weight problems and water retention benefit either from some of the physical elements, or from the combination of these and the moments of relaxation the programme results in.

PRIOR TO STARTING ANY PROGRAMME OF EXERCISE IT IS ADVISABLE TO CHECK WITH YOUR DOCTOR IF YOU THINK THERE IS ANY POSSIBILITY THAT IT MIGHT NOT BE RECOMMENDED FOR YOU.

Most people find a time of day that fits into their routine – home life, family commitments, work. It is important to try to find a time that you can allocate on a fairly regular basis. Remember what was said in the introduction about prioritising what is really important to you. If you want to feel better about yourself, and to have that fit body that will enable you to do the things you want in your later years, it is up to you to find the necessary time. Once you have started the programme and begun to feel the benefits, you will not find it difficult to find the time. This is because it will be so important to you to maintain this improvement.

Try to spread your exercise throughout the week rather than exercising on Monday, Tuesday and Wednesday, and then not for the rest of the week. This programme of exercise can be balanced by other types of exercise, which will be discussed in a later chapter, done on other days. Avoid doing your exercise after a heavy meal, when you will neither feel inclined nor able to move well (and are likely to feel sick through all the bending). Allow at least two hours to elapse before commencing.

1.6 Results

I strongly recommend you begin slowly, practise regularly, observe the gradual changes in your body and write it all down. I have given space (ppX–X) for this at the end of the book and would like you either to give yourself credit for your performance or at least record some sort of indication of how you feel. Do this simply by noting down how easy or difficult you found certain exercises, or how well or how poorly you felt having followed the programme on a particular day. Simply listing exercises that you find difficult and then noting when they no longer are difficult will give you an idea of the progress you are making. Believe me, it can vary – so from day to day be honest with yourself. Over time you will begin to realise some of the reasons for the variations, and as you feel fitter you will come to a better understanding of your body.

This can not be an overnight success story, but you will find the longer you exercise the better you feel and the calmer the body and mind become. You will also find small signs of progress occurring fairly quickly in relation to how easy some exercises become within a few attempts. It produces mental and physical strengths, also a marked feeling of well-being and harmony within yourself. You are possibly anxious to know how long it will take for this wonderful feeling to arrive.

My advice to you is to see what one week of exercising will do for you. Make a note of any change and then do the same for week two and so on. You will find it makes interesting reading as time goes on. Record not only the changes in how easy or difficult you find the exercises, but also how you feel generally and your attitude to other things in your life. For example, if you normally have little control over your will-power regarding what you eat, and you find that as you begin to feel better you begin to pay some attention to your dietary habits, this is a very significant happening, so it is important to make a record of this. Likewise, if you normally cannot be bothered to do certain things or regard them as chores, but due to feeling better or being more flexible and active discover that you no longer find these tasks overwhelming, record that fact too. These written records not only make interesting reading and help you to see your progress, they can also serve as a reminder and inspiration if you waver and fail to exercise and start to regress. Remember, this is your lifetime, body and mind you're working with. It is very special to you and the new you is your creation. It is quite an achievement, and comes at very little cost. It is your investment in the quality of the later years of your life.

On the days I don't work out I really miss it, but at least I go through the warm-up to keep my joints flexible. Even just a few of the stretching exercises performed when you get up in the morning, or when you get out of the shower or bath, will help to make you feel good, and will help to keep you in shape on the days when you cannot do the whole programme.

1.7 Frequency of working out

You may also be wondering how often you should work out. Four days out of seven is good. On the other days, as far as is possible, the warm-up should be done. If you plan to do three exercise sessions per week, in taking that decision you are making a positive step to improve your body, to give yourself a better chance of quality in later years. If you opt out of doing the programme, or if you too frequently miss doing one or two of your sessions during the week, you are making the decision to accept the quality of life and the body as it is, in its deteriorating state.

It is your choice when, how often and for how long you exercise; and it is always up to you to make that decision. This is another factor that makes the programme valuable, as you are always in control. You are taking charge of your body's needs, so that it feels good. Taking charge and making decisions, the results of which please you, is a very satisfying activity in itself. This does not mean that you require to be absolutely bound by the need to do the exercise every single day. Obsession with exercise is just as much a problem as not exercising at all. Try to get a balance between your commitment to it in order to improve your quality of life, fitting it in regularly without being obsessed about both it and all the other things you want to do with your time. A fitness programme that leaves no time for other activities is of little benefit.

It is true that we can all find the time to do the things that we really want to do. It is a question of priorities. Many of us are short of time for the wide range of activities that we try to fit in, or we spend so much time slouched in front of the television, mindlessly watching anything that's on, and this is a state of passive absorption. Sometimes we even sit around convinced we're exhausted and lacking the energy to move ourselves to more active and stimulating things. In reality we are not in control of our lives, we are needing to prioritise the things that are important for us in terms of *the quality of life that we want to lead.* In many cases this commences with getting our body into a state that it is ready and responsive, and where we feel good and in control. Only when this is the case can we go on to use our time in the ways we really want to, and so get the most from our later years.

Remember that we have this life only once. It is not a dress rehearsal. We don't have the chance to make a better life next time. We need to make sure that we are able to do what we want now or be working towards it. We need to make sure that our body is looked after so that it allows us to do the things we want to do in our later years, when there is much more time to devote to our interests. It is unfortunate that we appear to have little time to pursue these when there are work and family commitments when we're younger, fit and able. It seems almost a paradox that when time is granted us we are very much older and generally less able. That is a matter we hope this programme will help you to address. Make your later years a time of pleasure. Feel good, and not worn out. Participate in a whole range of things you have always wanted to do but have never had the time for. Be full of energy and able to get the most out of all that time now at your disposal.

If you feel passionate about wanting a new, poised, calm appearance, and a really fit body, then I think you know the answer. Keep at it until you reach your goal. By then you will be capable of adjusting the programme to suit your needs and commitments. You will know how often you need to exercise to feel good, and you will feel the lack of exercise when you miss a few days. That feeling alone will be enough to motivate you to keep going. Just knowing how much better you feel is a great inducement. I know you will like the new you in your life, so let's get started with the programme itself.

If you are in doubt about your ability to do the exercises, because of pre-existing health problems, consult your doctor before going any further.

Introducing the programme

WARM-UP

A significant part of the warm-up phase involves easy circling and stretching exercises to prepare the body for the main exercises that follow. To get the maximum benefit from circling and stretching it is important that the body temperature is raised slightly. The first few exercises are therefore fairly active in order to increase the heart rate and blood circulation, and raise the body temperature. These benefits enable you to do the subsequent exercises more fully and get a greater return from them.

The photographs are intended to guide you through the exercises and should be looked at carefully in conjunction with the text. They have been chosen to show the main positions or movements that you should be going through.

In the initial stages you will obviously have to spend quite a bit of time following the instructions in the text. However, once you have learned the exercises you will not need to refer to these details very often. There is a summary of the warm-up programme at the end of this section, to give you an easy-to-refer-to guide to follow, once you are familiar with the techniques involved.

Warm-up exercise 1: Marching

If fifty steps are too demanding to start with for 1(a), (b) or (c), begin with twenty and build up from that to fifty over two to three weeks. This is a five-part exercise, with less intense and more intense sections. New participants might find it easier to do this wearing shoes initially. The shoes need to be flat, soft and comfortable.

1(a) Start standing with feet slightly apart. Tramp steadily on the spot, fifty steps. Try to establish a brisk walking pace. Lift the feet just clear of the floor on every step. As the foot comes back onto the floor the toes should come down first, slightly before the heel. The knees should be slightly bent. The eyes should be looking forward focusing on something at about head-height.

1(b) Standing with feet slightly apart, body relaxed but straight, march on the spot, raising your knees to about hip-height for a count of fifty. Shake out legs and breathe deeply a few times.

1(c) Tramp easily on the spot again, just raising the feet off the floor for a count of fifty. This will allow a slight recovery from the previous high-knee-lift marching.

1 (a)

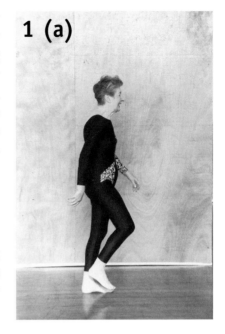

1 (b)

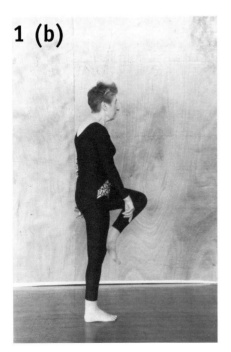

1 (c)

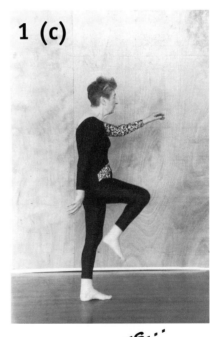

start the legs...
then bring in
the arms

1(d) Repeat the marching exercises 1(b), this time swinging the arms vigorously as well. Start the marching step first then add in the swinging of the arms. The right arm should be swung forward as the left knee is raised. You might find the arm-swinging difficult to start with, but keep persevering, trying to add the arms in for a short time. As you become more skilled or used to doing this, try to raise the arms to shoulder-level. Repeat for a count of fifty. Shake out arms and legs and breathe deeply a few times.

1(e) Repeat the tramp-easy exercise 1(c).

start with twenty, build up to fifty

Remember to breathe

deeply throughout

exercising

Warm up exercise 2: Shoulder shrugs

➤ Stand with the feet approximately a foot apart.

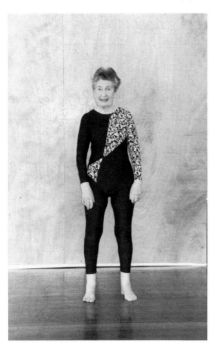

➤ Raise the shoulders towards the ears and rotate them in a forward direction five times. The sequence is: up to ears, forward, down as far as possible, back, then up.

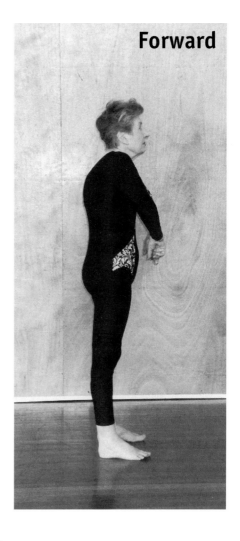

Forward

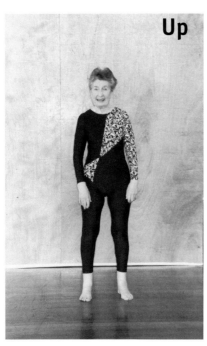

Up

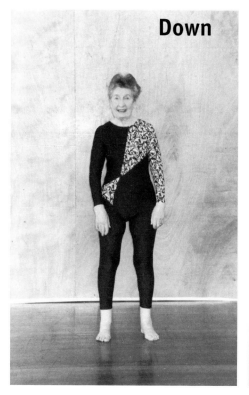

Down

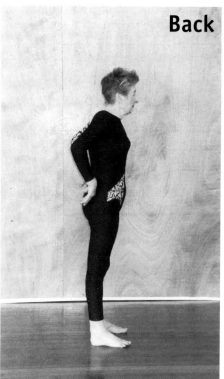

Back

➢ Remember to keep breathing steadily and regularly.

➢ Repeat the same shoulder movement rotating backwards five times. The sequence for backwards is up, backwards, down then forwards.

➢ Shake out shoulders, arms and hands like a rag doll. Shake out the legs too.

remember to keep your shoulders well down from your ears

Warm up exercise 3: Stretch

➤ Stand with feet about four inches apart, eyes open and focusing forward on something at about head-height. Throughout the exercise have the knees soft (relaxed), and very slightly bent rather than rigid.

➤ Slowly raise arms forwards and upwards until the hands are above your head. Breathe in deeply as you move the arms upwards.

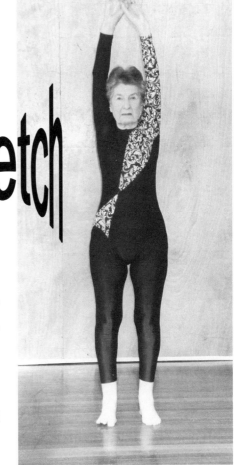

➤ In this upright stretched position raise the chest and draw the ribs upwards away from the hips. Feel there is a space between the ribs and the hips. Feel you are growing taller.

➤ Start moving downwards and forwards by lowering the arms. As the arms pass the head bring the chin forward onto the chest.

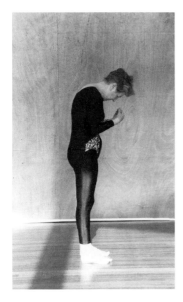

➤ Curl the shoulders, upper back, waist region and then bend at the hips to allow the arms to reach forward towards the floor. Breathe out as you descend.

➤ Stay in this relaxed position for a count of ten. Keep your eyes open to assist your balance.

➤ Slowly return to an upright position by uncurling, Stretch up through the hips, spine, shoulders and then the head. The arms should move upwards with the hands being drawn up the body, past the shoulders and finally stretched up overhead. Breathe in as you move upwards.

➤ Repeat twice more. Shake out arms and legs each time.

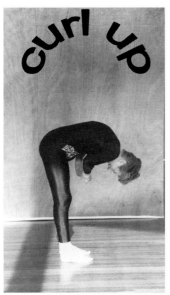

curl up

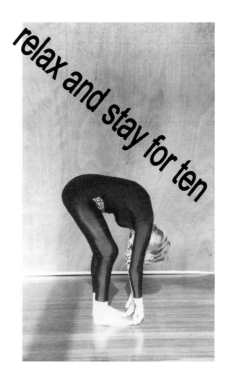

relax and stay for ten

An easier version for beginners is following the upward stretch, bend the knees, curl down over the knees and grasp behind the knees. Keep the feet flat on the floor. In that position, round the back, pushing it slightly upwards.

4(a) Chin stretches

Stand with the feet approximately one foot apart, hands relaxed by your side. The head should be in an upright position with the eyes focusing forward on something at about head-height.

Imagine you are sliding your chin forward along a shelf just in front of you.

Reach as far forward as you can, then drop the head down to bring the chin onto the chest.

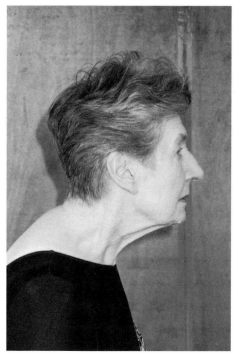

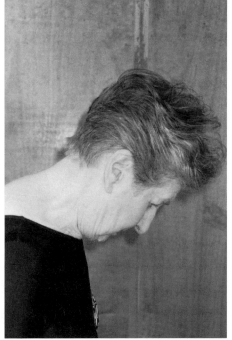

Hold for a count of ten.

Repeat twice more then relax.

Hold for a count of ten. Repeat.

4(b) Neck rolls

From the upright position turn the head so that you are looking upwards over your right shoulder.

Drop the chin towards the shoulder, then move the chin across the chest towards the left shoulder.

Lift the head so that you are looking upward over your left shoulder.

Repeat five times.

Do not take the head backwards in this exercise.

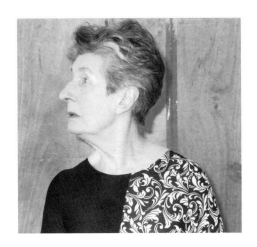

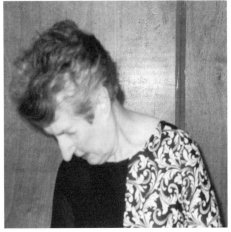

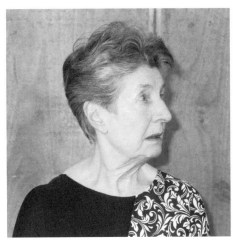

all exercises should be smooth and rhythmic, never jerky

Warm-up exercise 5: Left and right side stretch

➤ Stand with the feet shoulder-width apart.

➤ Raise arms sideways and upward to shoulder-level.

➤ Very slowly, bend the body to the right side and bring the right arm down by the side of your right leg. Keep the legs slightly bent and reach only as far as you can without bending the body forwards.

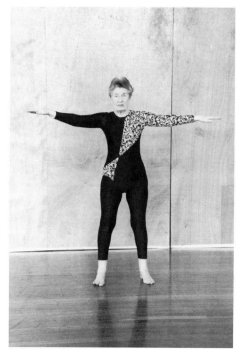

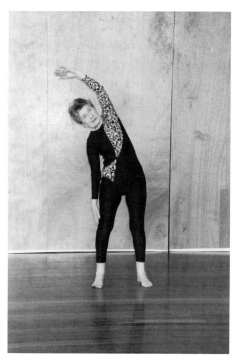

➤ Your left arm continues to move towards the left side of the head so that the left side of the body is stretched.

➤ Hold for a count of ten.

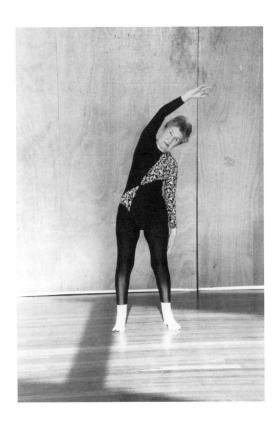

➢ In a rhythmic movement return to the starting position to repeat on the other side.

➢ Maintain regular breathing. Do this by breathing in on the upward movements and breathing out on the downward movements.

➢ Repeat twice more on each side.

➢ Shake out arms and legs.

If you follow the instructions for each exercise you should never suffer from exhaustion or injury.

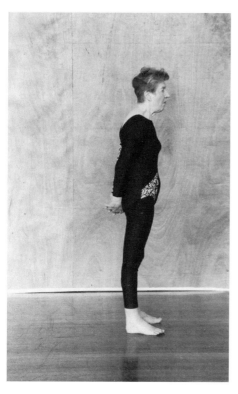

➤ Stand with feet approximately four inches apart.

➤ Firmly clasp your hands behind your back with the palms facing upwards.

➤ Press the hands down towards the hips as if you are going to sit on your hands.

➤ Hold for a count of ten.

➤ Release the hands gently. Do not do this suddenly.

➤ Shake out hands, arms and legs.

at the end of the exercise shake out hands, arms and legs

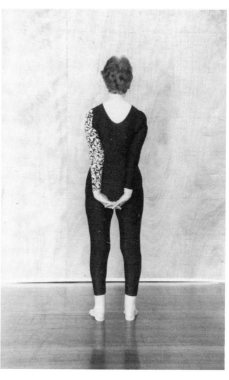

Warm-up exercise 7: Twist

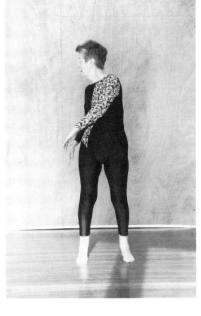

➤ Stand with feet approximately hip-width apart, arms hanging loosely by your side. The knees should be slightly bent.

➤ Twist your body right and left rhythmically, allowing the arms to swing easily as you twist.

➤ Twist at the waist only. The hips should remain facing squarely forwards. Keep the knees slightly bent.

➤ The head should turn in the same direction as the shoulders.

➤ Repeat ten times.

➤ Do not allow this exercise to become too fast as you swing from side to side, as you will lose the effective twisting action.

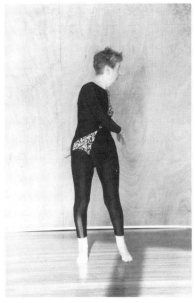

➤ Shake out arms and legs.

Question I find it difficult to keep my hips facing squarely forward while twisting. What can I do to improve it?

Answer If you have difficulty keeping the hips from rotating try doing the exercise without letting the arms swing, so that you are really concentrating on the movement at a slow pace. You can also try concentrating on the hip on the side to which you are twisting the shoulders, i.e. as you twist the shoulders to the right push the right hip forward just as you reach the point of the maximum twist.

Warm-up exercise 8: Pendulum

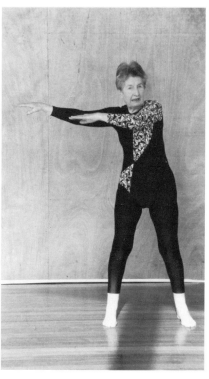

➤ Stand upright with the feet approximately two feet apart.

➤ Lift both arms to shoulder-level, stretching towards the right.

➤ Bend at the ankles, knees and hips; let the arms drop down to sweep across in front of the body. The hands should reach down to about the knees as they pass in front.

Initially you may wish to start with eight or ten repeats and build up to twenty.

➤ Extend the ankles, knees and hips as the arms rise towards the other side so that they finish at shoulder-level stretched towards the left.

➤ Keep the feet flat on the floor throughout the exercise.

➤ Maintain regular breathing throughout.

➤ Repeat twenty times.

➤ Try to establish an easy regular rhythm.

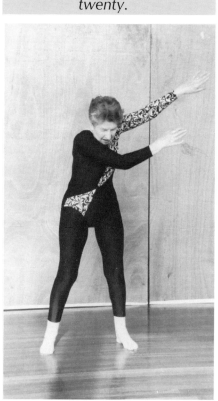

Warm-up exercise 9: Stepping

This is a six-part exercise with some less intense and some more intense parts.

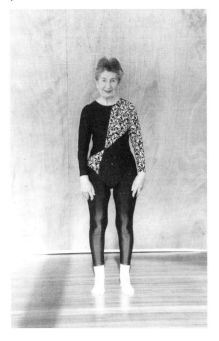

9(a) Stepping forward

Start standing with the feet about six inches apart.

Keeping the weight on the left foot, place the right heel on the ground about ten inches forward.

Bring the right foot back to its original place.

Repeat with the left foot. Keeping the weight on the right foot place the left heel on the ground about ten inches forward.

Bring the left foot back to its original place.

Repeat for thirty steps in total.

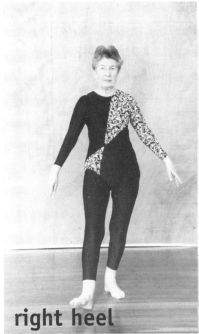

right heel

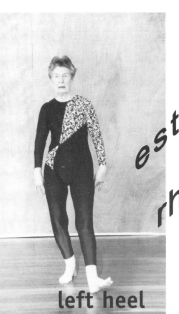

left heel

establish a rhythm

9(b) Stepping forward with elbow bending

This a repeat of the above exercise, 9(a), with the addition of elbow bending.

Start the stepping action first and then bring in the arm movement. The arms bend at the elbow bringing the hands up towards the shoulders. This movement occurs each time the heel is placed on the ground.

Repeat for thirty steps. If thirty steps are too demanding to start with begin with fifteen and build up to thirty over a week or two.

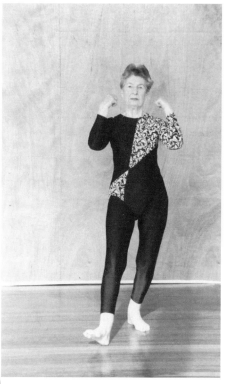

start with the feet, then bring in the arms

9(c) Sideways stepping

Starting with the feet together, keep the weight on the right foot and stretch the left foot out to the side as if to take a step to the left.

Bring the left foot back to its original place.

Repeat to the right. Keeping the weight on the left foot stretch the right foot out to the side as if to take a sideways step.

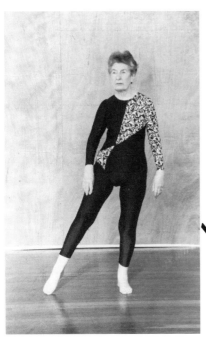

Return the right foot to the starting position.

Repeat for a total of thirty steps.

left foot out... back together... right

9(d) Sideways stepping with arm swinging

Repeat the above exercise, 9(c), with sideways arm swinging. Start the side stepping exercise and then bring in the arm movement. Each time a foot stretches to the side both arms swing out from the sides. As the feet come together the arms return to the sides. Try to raise the arms up to shoulder-level.

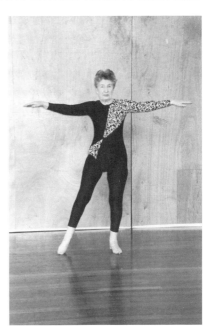

Repeat for thirty steps. If you find this too demanding to start with, begin with fifteen steps and gradually increase to thirty over a week or two.

as above—plus— arms swing out with each foot

9(e) Backward stepping

Starting with the feet about hip-width apart, keeping the weight on the right foot, move the left foot back to place the toes on the floor about ten inches behind.

Return the foot to the original position.

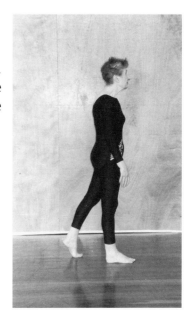

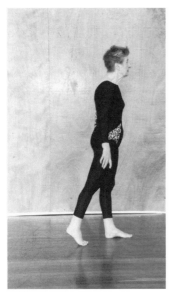

Keep the weight on the left foot and move the right foot back to place the toes on the floor about ten inches behind.

Return the foot to the original position

Repeat for thirty steps.

9(f) Backward stepping with forward arm swinging

Repeat the above exercise, 9(e), with forward arm swinging.

Start the stepping action and then bring in the arm movement so that the arms swing forward each time a leg moves back.

The arms should swing up to shoulder-level.

Repeat for thirty steps. If necessary start with fifteen and increase to thirty over a period of two weeks.

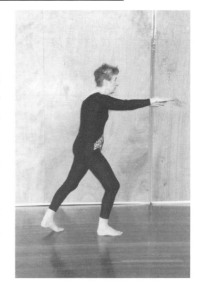

Question

I have great difficulty co-ordinating the movements of the arms with the legs. This is the reason I stopped going to aerobics – I could not get the feet and the arms co-ordinated. Is there anything I can do to solve the problem, or is this another activity that I just cannot do?

Answer

It really does not matter if you are not very good at co-ordinating the arms and legs. The reason for using both is that when you use the arms as well as the legs the increased activity gets you much warmer and it makes significantly more demands on the heart and lungs to circulate more oxygen-carrying blood around the body. Both these factors are important in preparing the body for exercise. As an alternative you could do more of the basic stepping without the arm action and you could try to increase the pace of it to make it more demanding. You can also keep having a short try at using the arms. Always start the legs first, and then bring in the arms once you have the rhythm of the legs established. In time you will manage these basic variations.

Even if you're tempted, _do not_ close your eyes in any of the standing exercises.

If your sense of balance is poor, do not keep your feet close together in standing exercises.

Warm-up exercise 10: Press-up standing

➤ Use a wall or closed door for this exercise.

➤ Stand with feet together and a straight-arm's distance from the wall or door.

➤ Place your hands on the wall or door in front of your forehead with the fingertips pointing towards each other and touching. An easier position of the hands for you, if you are just beginning the programme, is to place them with the fingers pointing upwards and each hand in front of the shoulder.

➤ Very slowly bend the elbows and rest your forehead on your hands. The body should be in a straight line. (If the fingers are pointing upwards the head will be between the hands.)

➤ Rest your forehead on your hands for a count of ten then slowly push back straightening the arms to return to a standing position.

➤ Maintain regular breathing throughout.

➤ Repeat twice more.

➤ Shake out arms and legs.

breathe regularly!

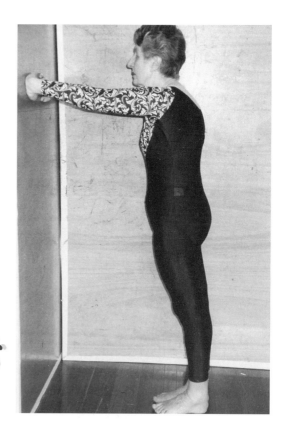

28

Warm-up exercise 11: Tree

If your balance is poor it is quite acceptable to use the other hand to hold on to a chair or wall for support. It may be that you just need to be by the wall with only the slightest touch on it for support. Concentration is required for this exercise.

➢ Stand with feet together.

➢ Bend knee of right leg, so that the foot moves back and up.

➢ Reach back with the right hand, catch the ankle and draw the foot in towards the buttocks. The supporting leg *must be kept straight*. The knee of the bent leg should be touching the straight leg.

use the wall or a chair

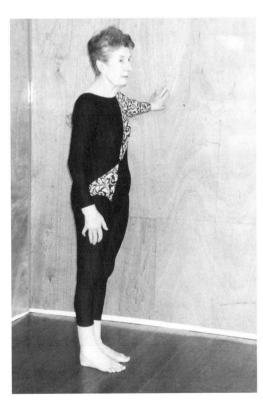

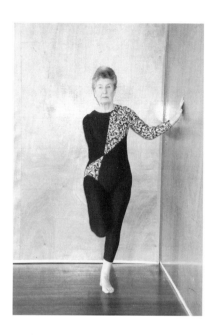

> Your eyes should be focused forward on something at about head-height.

> Maintain regular breathing.

> Initially use a chair or the wall for support. As your control of this posture improves try to use the free arm stretched out to the side for balance. Only when skilled at this exercise should you try raising the free arm above the head. This brings in the element of balance as well as the stretching of the muscle at the front of the thigh.

> Hold for a count of ten.

> Repeat on left side.

Keep those knees together.

Feel the stretch

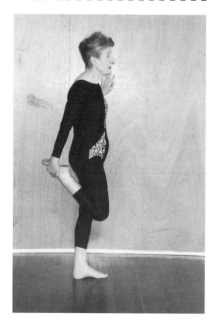

the tree

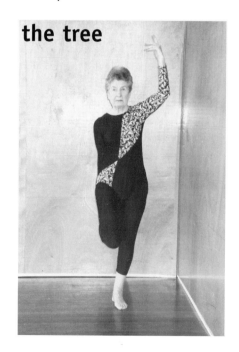

Question

I have great difficulty getting hold of my ankle behind me. I'm not sure whether it is the lifting up of the lower leg backwards or the reaching down to find my ankle that's the problem. I'm so nearly overbalancing that I cannot concentrate on finding my foot to get hold of. Any ideas for making it easier?

Question

I find that either I cannot hold the bent leg with its knee beside the straight leg or, if I do, it is extremely painful down the front of my thigh. Am I doing something wrong?

> **Remember that it takes time to achieve some of the exercises... and still more time to do them really well.**

Answer

First, use a chair or wall to hold onto. There is no reason to struggle in a state of imbalance. Even some of the young and very fit people find balance on one foot difficult. Second, start by raising your knee in front of you and taking hold of the ankle there, then draw the leg behind you to continue the exercise.

Answer

This exercise is about stretching the muscle on the front of the thigh. To do the exercise correctly you should keep the bent knee beside the straight leg and I advise you to try to get that part correct. In the initial attempts do not try to pull your foot up too close to your buttocks at the back and do not attempt to straighten the hip too much, i.e., the movement of pushing the hip forward as you draw the foot back. These slight adjustments in the initial stages will reduce the stretch on the muscle on the front of the thigh that you are finding painful. Once you are more familiar with the exercise you can gradually pull the foot up closer to the buttocks and straighten the hip joint fully.

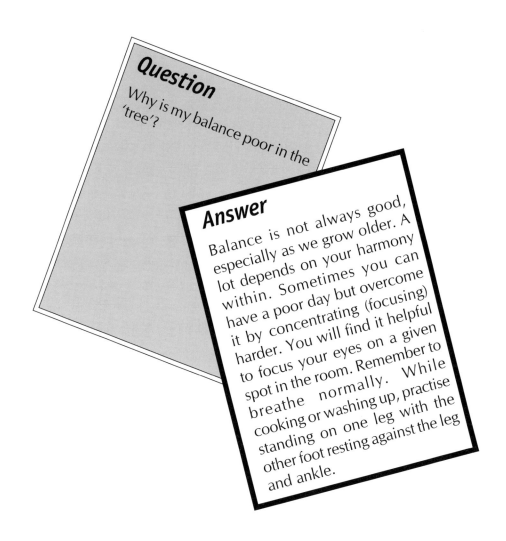

Question

Why is my balance poor in the 'tree'?

Answer

Balance is not always good, especially as we grow older. A lot depends on your harmony within. Sometimes you can have a poor day but overcome it by concentrating (focusing) harder. You will find it helpful to focus your eyes on a given spot in the room. Remember to breathe normally. While cooking or washing up, practise standing on one leg with the other foot resting against the leg and ankle.

Warm-up exercise 12: Hamstring and calf stretch

→ Stand upright with feet hip-width apart.

→ Place the left heel on the floor about twelve inches forward with the toes as far off the floor as possible.

→ Keep the body-weight back over the bent right leg.

→ Place the hands above the knee of the bent back leg.

➤ Feel the stretch in the muscles (hamstrings and calf) at the back of the straight leg.

➤ Hold for a count of ten.

➤ Release slowly.

➤ Repeat on the other side.

➤ Repeat twice more on either side.

➤ Shake out arms and legs.

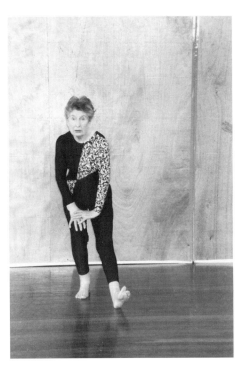

Question

I do not really feel any stretch when I am doing this exercise. What am I doing wrong?

Answer

If you are not feeling a stretch in the muscle at the back of the straight leg there are generally two possible reasons. Make sure that you are 'sitting back' into the movement with your weight firmly over the bent leg. Also make sure that you have the toes of the straight leg up off the floor, i.e., really pulled up towards the knee. This increases the stretch significantly.

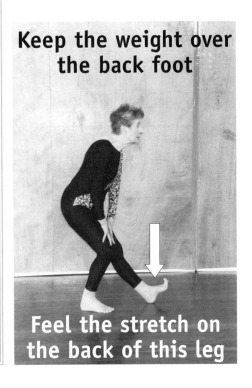

Keep the weight over the back foot

Feel the stretch on the back of this leg

Target Areas

This table summarises the warm-up exercises and their main target areas.

Exercise	Target Area
1 Marching	General temperature raiser
2 Shoulder shrug	Shoulder area joints and muscles
3 Stretch	Postural alignment. Movement of the spine
4 Chin stretch and neck rolls	Neck joints and muscles
5 Left and right side stretches	Spine sideways flexion
6 Sit on hands	Shoulder extension
7 Twist	Spine rotation
8 Pendulum	General temperature raiser and all joints and muscles
9 Stepping variations	General temperature raiser
10 Press-up standing	Elbow flexors/extensors
11 Tree	Hip and knee joints, muscles of the hip/knee
12 Hamstrings/calf stretch	Hamstrings/calf muscles

It is important to begin to develop an understanding (without going into great depth on the scientific aspects) of what you are doing to your body. The series of warm-up exercises has attempted to raise the body's temperature slightly so that all your joints and muscles will function with maximum efficiency. Then it has taken the muscle groups around each joint of the body and stretched them through their normal range of movement.

You will notice I keep telling you to shake out arms and legs and to breathe normally. Both are extremely important and will make sure of the least discomfort and exhaustion. The next series of positions is more demanding and consists of the important exercises to improve the physical condition of the body, and that will have the revitalising and rejuvenating effect.

Summary of the warm-up programme

This is intended to serve as a quick reference guide once you know the techniques of the warm-up exercises, and is put in to remind you of what comes next in the warm-up, how many repeats to do and so on.

Marching	Tramp for fifty High knee march for fifty Tramp for fifty March with arms swinging for fifty Tramp for fifty
Shoulder shrugs	Forwards for five/backwards for five
Stretch	Repeat three times
Chin stretch and neck rolls	Chin stretches three times Neck rolls five times
Left and right side stretch	Three times to each side

Sit on hands	Once
Twist	Repeat ten times
Pendulum	Repeat twenty times
Stepping variations	Forward thirty steps Forward plus elbow bending, thirty steps Sideways stepping, thirty steps Sideways stepping/arms swinging for thirty steps Backward thirty steps Backward stepping/forward arm swings for thirty steps
Press-up standing	Repeat three times
Tree	Once on each leg
Hamstring/calf stretch	Three times on each side

The main exercises

Positions and benefits

If you are not very fit or if you are over-weight I suggest you have some form of support close to you to give you confidence – a strong chair is ideal. You require a travel rug or mat and a small thin cushion for your head.

Put your cushion at the end of your mat where you will place your head and lie down in a straight line. Adjust your cushion until the back of your skull rests in its centre. Many people do not require a cushion, but the older you are the more likely you are to need this comfort.

This section includes some of the questions that people sometimes raise about exercises, and about their progress or problems with some of the exercises in the early stages. Hopefully these will reassure you that you are experiencing a similar learning process to other people, and that there are many questions that occur during such a programme of activity. These are, however, relatively minor points, and I hope I have included all the items that are of concern to you, either within the instruction text for each exercise or within the questions.

Again, as with the warm-up photographs, the ones in this section are intended as a guide. It is recommended that you look at them carefully as they provide a good model of the exercise being performed by an older person. They have been selected to show the key points or positions within each exercise, and as such, studied together with the text, they should give you a clear idea of the movement you are attempting.

Exercise 1: Long stretch and sit-up

Benefit: strengthens and tones abdominal muscles and stretches the hamstring muscles.

Sit on the floor with the legs outstretched and the toes turned up.

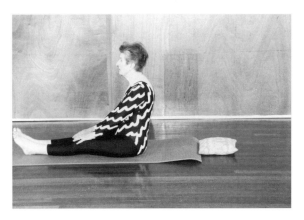

Rest the hands on your knees.

Lie back to the floor. Lie down by aiming to put the small of the back on the floor first, then the shoulder blades, then the neck, and then the head. Slide the hands up the thighs as you lie down.

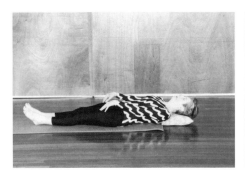 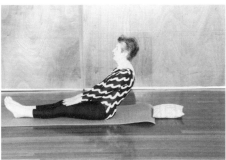

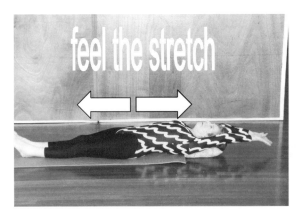

feel the stretch

Stretch both arms beyond the head until the hands touch the floor. As you reach this position you should feel a stretch between the rib cage and the hips.

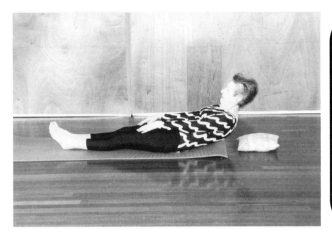

raise the head...
then the neck...
then the
shoulders...
then the upper
back

Return the hands to the thighs and start to raise the body back to the sitting position.

The hands should remain in contact with the thighs as they slide forward. The return to the sitting position should be done by first raising the head off the floor, then the neck, then the shoulder blades, then the small of the back.

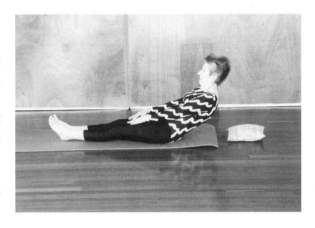

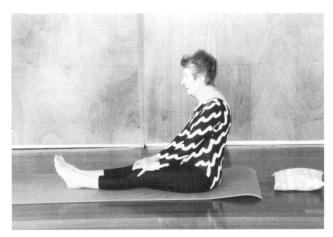

Repeat three times.

Hold for a count of ten.

Maintain regular breathing.

Exercise 2: Forward bend sitting

Benefit: stretches the hamstring muscles.

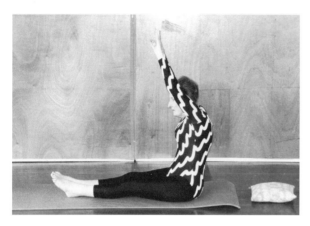

Sit on the floor with the legs outstretched and the toes turned up.

Slowly raise both arms above your head.

Feel the stretch between the rib cage and the hips.

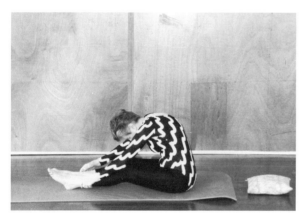

Bend at the hips then bring the chest towards the knees. Bring the arms to rest as far down the legs as possible. If you are a beginner in the programme reach as far forward as possible and hold on to the legs to stabilise yourself, and to help achieve the stretch of the back postural muscles.

Stop where it is comfortable, feeling a stretch in the muscles of the back of the thigh (the hamstrings), and hold that position for a count of ten.

Return to the upright sitting position.

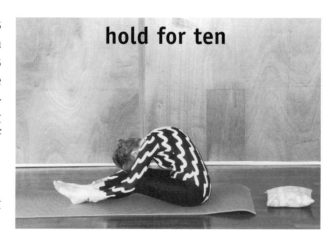

hold for ten

Repeat twice more without resting.

Do this smoothly without jerking or bouncing and keeping the outstretched legs flat on the floor.

Question

Why am I not doing very well at the forward bend?

Further helpful hints

When you assume the sitting position raise your rib cage as far away from your upper thighs as you can. This helps ensure that you are sitting correctly. As you start the stretch-forward part of the movement, first try to put the lower abdomen against the upper thighs, then the lower edge of the rib cage with the upper chest area coming forward last. Eventually, when bending forward, you should be able to place the upper body flat against the thighs.

Answer

It may be that you are sitting on the base of your spine rather than sitting upright. You should feel that you are sitting with your weight on your two seat bones, almost on the back of your thighs.

Come out of each exercise the way you went in, never collapse in a heap.

Exercise 3: Breathing through the nose only

Benefit: Increases circulation of oxygen. Improves breathing habits.

Lie flat on the back, trying to press the small of the back against the floor. Adjust your position until you feel comfortable, but ensuring that the small of the back is as close to the floor as possible. Check that the chin is slightly tucked in, ensuring that it is not higher than the forehead. This is an exercise where the use of a small cushion might be necessary to ensure the correct head position.

Take three deep breaths before starting the main breathing exercise.

To inhale, start your breathing by allowing the abdomen to extend. This allows the lower areas of the lungs to expand. Then the rib cage and upper chest area should expand as they fill with air.

Inhale, through the nostrils only, as fully as possible.

To exhale, slowly breathe out by contracting the muscles of the abdomen.

Exhale, through the nostrils only, as fully as possible.

Repeat the exercise five times, breathing through both nostrils.

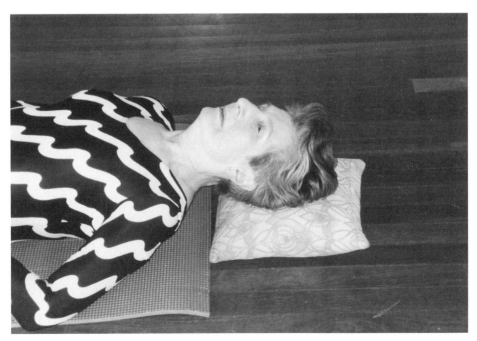

Exercise 4: Alternate leg stretch

Benefit: Mobility of the legs. Rejuvenates the spine by making it strong and supple.

Sit on the floor, legs outstretched, back straight.

Bend the left knee. Carefully lift the left foot and place its sole to the top of the inside right thigh. If you cannot get your foot to the top of the thigh just place it as far up the leg as you can (as in the photo).

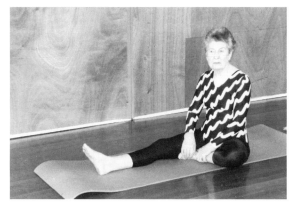

Raise both arms with the elbows bent and the hands clasped.

Breathe in raising the rib cage before stretching forward to move the chest towards the knee. Grasp the ankle and then let the head drop forward towards the knee. If you cannot reach the ankle grasp as far down the legs as you can.

Stop while still comfortable but feeling a stretch in the hamstring muscle on the back of the thigh.

Hold the position for a count of ten. Straighten up very slowly and repeat on the other side.

Repeat twice more to each side. (Do this exercise very slowly. Remember to breathe normally and keep the long leg straight.)

Take three deep breaths before proceeding to the next exercise.

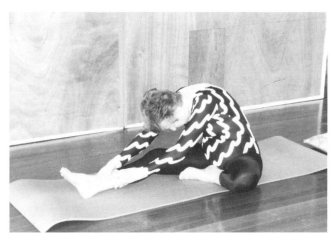

Question Why do I remain very stiff in the alternate leg stretch exercise?

Answer Make sure that you are sitting up straight. If the long thigh muscle is tight it will take quite a lot of time to stretch it out. It will become easier and will stretch over time but do not force it. Keep practising sitting cross-legged. Putting your small head-cushion under your seat is helpful.

Keep practising sitting cross-legged!

Exercise 5: Hip rotation

Benefit: Keep hip joints flexible.

Lie stretched out on your back.

Bring the knees up towards the chest.

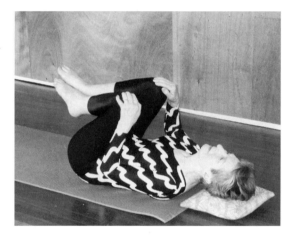

With one hand firmly clasping each knee, rotate both hip joints in a circular motion. The knees should come apart, then away from you, then together, then towards you.

Turn first in one direction and then in the other.

Do ten rotations each way. This exercise should be done rhythmically.

Take three deep breaths before proceeding to the next exercise.

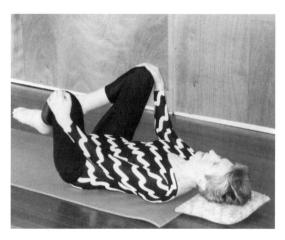

Exercise 6: Rock-'n'-roll

Benefit: Builds confidence for working on the floor. Good all-round exercise and generally enjoyed by most people.

Sit on the floor with knees bent.

Clasp hands very firmly under the knees.

Bring the head forward onto the knees and keep the body in a compact rounded shape.

In this position rock backwards and forwards ten times.

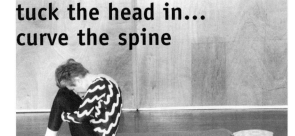

**tuck the head in...
curve the spine**

Once you become used to the exercise you should go far enough back so that the back of the head touches the floor.

Make sure your head touches your knees as you come forward.

Keep the spine curved, so that the body rocks easily. This will help maintain the momentum. The continuous rhythm helps you return to the forward sitting position again.

Take three deep breaths before proceeding to the next exercise.

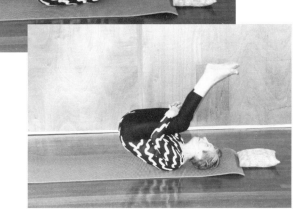

Answer You must be in the upright sitting position, the hands must be very firmly locked. A matter of practice, this one, but most people enjoy this exercise.

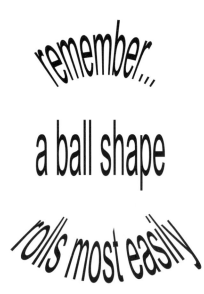

remember...

a ball shape

rolls most easily

Exercise 7:

Back massage/side rock

Benefit: Builds confidence in working on the floor.

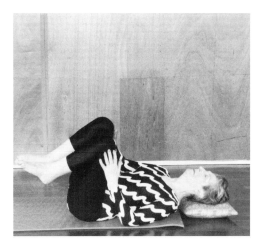

➤ Sit on the floor, knees bent with a hand placed around each knee.

➤ Lie back in this position, keeping hold of the bent knees, until the back of the head is on the floor. Use small pillow if desired.

➤ Slowly and gently rock from side to side.

➤ Repeat ten times. (Use your elbows for balance if you feel you are rolling over.)

➤ Take three deep breaths before proceeding to the next exercise.

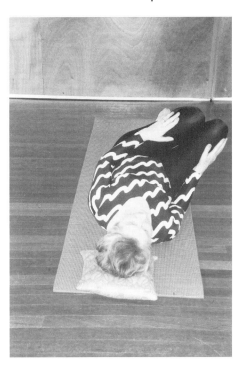

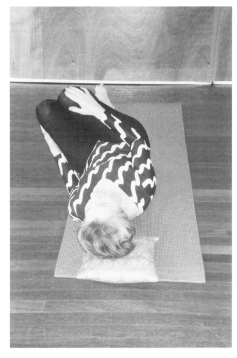

Exercise 8: Forehead to knee

Benefit: Strengthens upper back and neck.

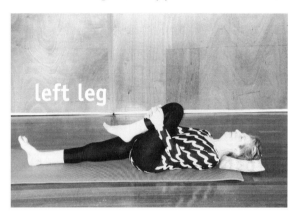

→ Lie on the floor, flat on the back.

→ Raise one knee towards the chest.

→ Clasp both hands around the knee and raise the head and shoulders just off the floor.

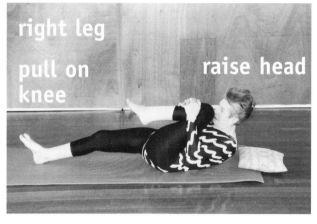

→ Pull the knee in towards the head until it touches the nose.

→ Release gently to return to the lying position.

→ Repeat with the other leg bent.

→ Repeat with both legs raised at the same time.

→ Repeat left leg, right leg and both legs three times each.

→ Take three deep breaths before proceeding to the next exercise.

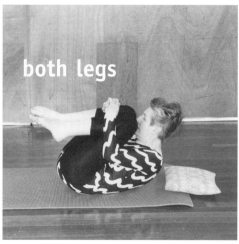

Exercise 9: Cross legged: elbow to knee rotations

Benefit: Reduces the waist-line and tones up abdominal muscles.

➤ Sit up straight in a cross-legged position.

➤ Clasp the hands behind the head so that the elbow points out left and right.

➤ Bring the right elbow down as near as possible to the left knee.

➤ Return to the upright sitting position.

➤ Repeat, bringing left elbow to right knee.

➤ Repeat five times on each side. (This is a form of twist.)

➤ Take three deep breaths before proceeding to the next exercise.

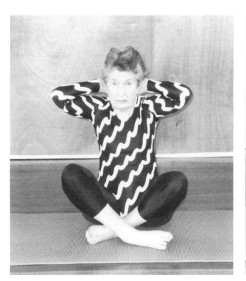 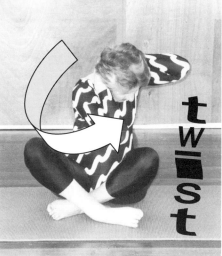

If you follow the instructions for each exercise you should never suffer from exhaustion or injury.

Exercise 10: Twist lying down

Benefit: A demanding exercise with great rewards. It firms the abdominal area and helps to alleviate backache. It helps mobility in so many areas that it is worth working at.

Stretch out on the floor flat on the back with the arms raised to shoulder-level.

Raise both knees towards the chest.

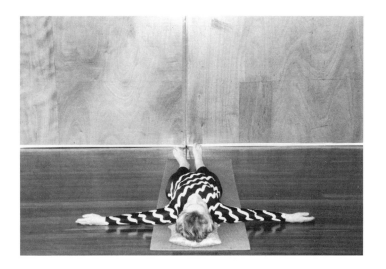

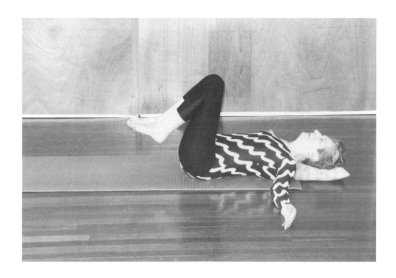

Keeping the knees bent and together, lower the knees to the floor, first to the left-hand side, then to the right-hand side. The head should turn to the opposite side to the bent knees.

In order to assist you in bringing the legs back to the centre position you may find it helpful to press the elbow into the floor on the lifting side.

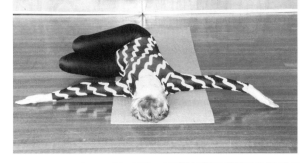

knees towards left hand

twist left, twist right

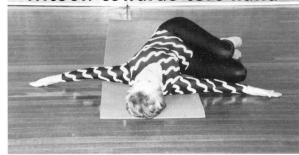

knees towards right hand ...look towards left hand

Hold for a count of ten on each side.

Repeat three times to each side.

Slowly raise knees back to the centre and lower the legs to the floor.

Take five deep breaths before proceeding to the next exercise.

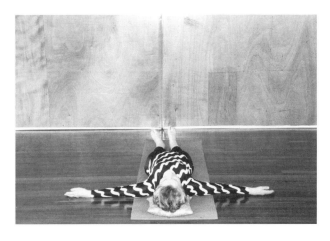

Exercise 11: Twist sitting up

Benefit: General spinal mobility, balance and poise.

⮑ Start in a sitting position with the legs stretched out on the floor. Bend the right knee to bring the foot up towards the groin. Place the right foot under the left thigh.

⮑ Lift the left leg over the right knee placing the left foot flat on the floor.

⮑ Shuffle round in this position until you feel really comfortable and stable. You should be sitting with your weight more forward than backward.

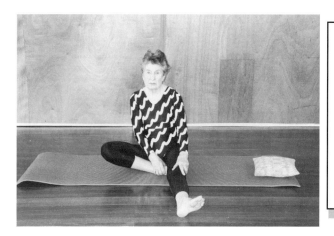

find a stable sitting position

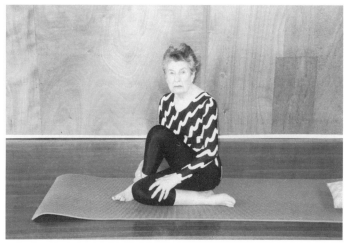

⊃ Place the right arm around the left knee.

⊃ Place your left hand behind you for support.

⊃ Twist your upper body towards the left. At the same time, using your right arm, pull the left knee across towards the right side of the body.

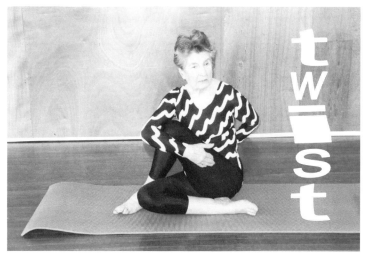

⊃ Place the supporting left hand across the back at waist-level. If you cannot manage this stage then initially maintain the hand on the floor to aid your balance.

⊃ Hold for a count of ten.

⊃ Gently release the hold and then repeat to the other side.

⊃ Take five deep breaths before progressing to the next exercise.

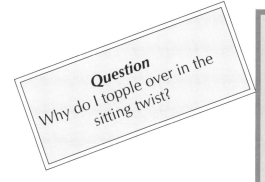

Question
Why do I topple over in the sitting twist?

Answer You are not balanced in your sitting position. Once the legs are crossed, shift around until you feel stable. Ensure that you are sitting more on the back of your thighs rather than on the back of your hips. Sit up straight.

Exercise 12: Cobra

Benefit: Exercises the spine and tones up the hip muscles.

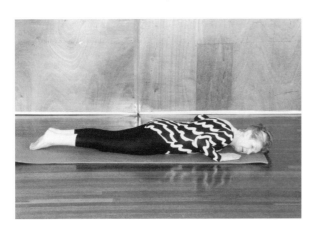

Lie flat on the front then place the hands one under each shoulder with the fingers pointing forwards.

Rest your head to one side. The head should have the chin slightly towards the chest, rather than the neck extended.

When you feel comfortable, push up on your hands to raise yourself up. Push up until the arms are straight.

Hold for a count of ten.

Bend the arms to lower the body until the pubic bone touches the floor. The shoulders, head and the back will be slightly arched. Keep the ears as far away from the shoulders as possible.

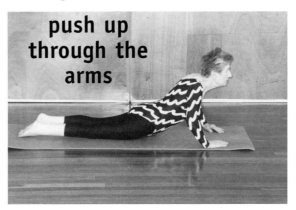

push up through the arms

Come out of this position very slowly by further bending the arm and lower the body to the floor.

Take five deep breaths before proceeding to the next exercise.

Question
Why do I find the cobra exercise a strain on my wrists?

Answer When you lie on your front to commence the cobra, go down on your forearms and hands. This takes the weight better, then push up onto your hands. This is an exercise where you must concentrate on keeping the shoulders away from the ears.

Exercise 13: The cat

Benefit: Helps to make the spine supple.

➤ Kneel and place the hands on the floor, shoulder-width apart, in front of the knees. Hands should be vertically below the shoulders.

➤ Push the spine upwards as far as you can, drawing the abdomen in and dropping the head between the arms as you do so.

➤ Hold for a count of five.

➤ Lower the back into the horizontal position again. In this position the eyes should be looking downwards towards the fingers.

➤ Repeat five times.

➤ Take five deep breaths before proceeding to the next exercise.

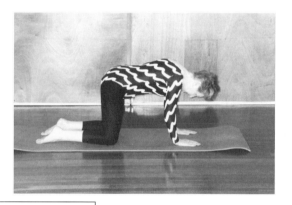

Remember you should have warmed up before attempting these kinds of exercises.

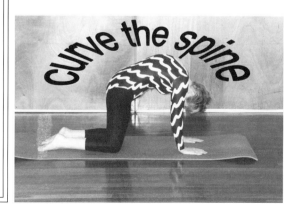

curve the spine

Exercise 14: Cat stretch

Benefit: Tones the hip muscles.

➤ Kneel and place the hands on the floor, shoulder-width apart, in front of the knees. Hands should be vertically below the shoulders.

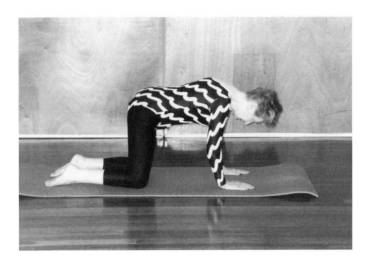

➤ Extend the right leg behind the body, toe pointing to the floor.

➤ Bring the bent knee of the right leg towards the chest as far as possible and bring the head down to meet the knee.

➤ Hold for a count of five.

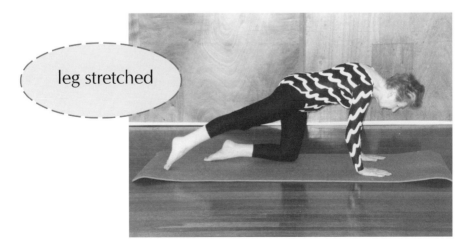

leg stretched

➤ Extend the right leg behind the body again with the foot raised off the floor and level with the body.

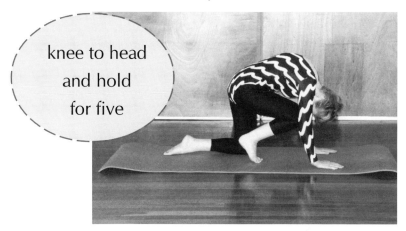

knee to head
and hold
for five

➤ Hold for a count of five.

➤ Return to the starting position and repeat the exercise with the left leg.

➤ Repeat the whole exercise twice more.

➤ Take five deep breaths before proceeding to the next exercise.

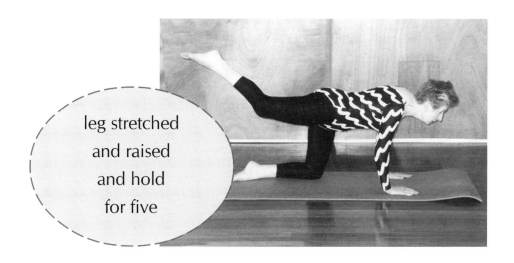

leg stretched
and raised
and hold
for five

Exercise 15: Pose of a child

Benefit: Wonderfully relaxing, improves circulation.

➡ Kneel on the floor keeping the legs together.

➡ Sit back on the heels.

➡ Bring the head forward and rest the forehead on the floor with your chest and abdomen lying along the thighs.

➡ The arms should be in a relaxed position and lying on the floor, beside the lower legs, with the hands palm up, beside the feet.

➡ Go into this position very slowly and come out of it just as slowly.

➡ Hold the position for a count of twenty.

➡ Return to the kneeling position.

➡ Repeat twice more.

➡ Take three deep breaths before proceeding to the next exercise.

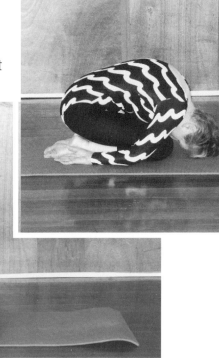

Exercise 16: Head to floor

Benefit: Allows a surge of blood to the brain. This is quite an advanced exercise and it should be left out for the first few weeks until you feel the benefits of the programme in terms of muscle strength. In the first few weeks concentrate on the pose of a child (previous exercise) instead.

➡ Kneel on the floor with the legs and feet slightly apart.

➡ Place the hands on the floor shoulder-width apart.

➡ Bend the arms and place the top of the head on the floor.

➡ Once you feel stable take the hands off the floor and clasp them behind the hips.

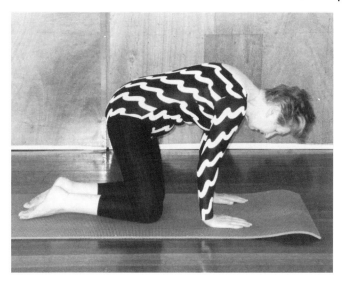

This is quite an advanced exercise and it should be left out for the first few weeks.

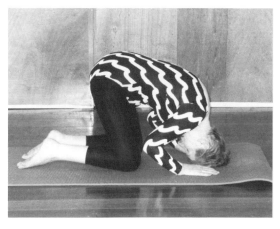

➡ Raise your hands as high as possible towards the vertical position behind you.

➡ Hold for a count of ten.

➡ Very slowly lower the hands and replace them on the floor.

➡ Very slowly return to the upright kneeling position.

➡ Repeat the exercise once more.

➡ Take three deep breaths before proceeding to the next exercise.

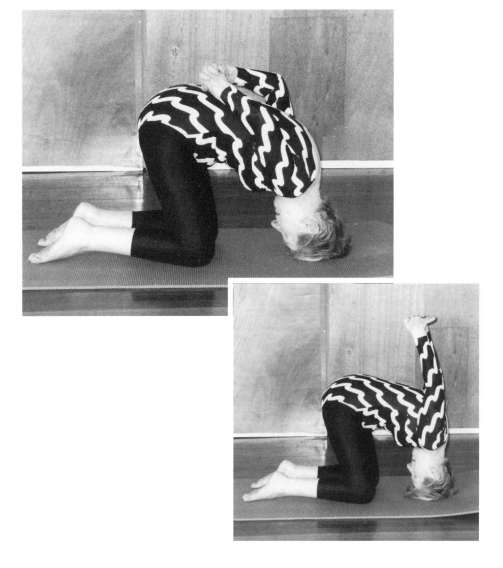

Exercise 17: Pelvic stretch

Benefit: Provides a good stretch of the front of the body and thighs. However in beginners who have not undertaken much exercise, problems might be experienced in assuming the kneeling position with the body-weight back over the feet. If this proves to be an uncomfortable position for you, concentrate on the cobra (exercise twelve) instead. Kneel on the floor with legs together.

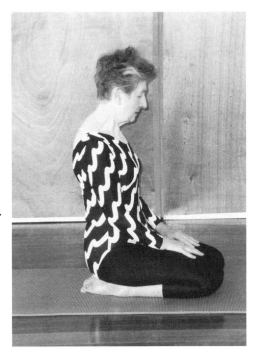

➥ Sit back on the heels and with the hands and arms stretched out behind you, place the palms of the hands on the floor.

➥ The arms must be straight.

➥ Raise the hips off the feet and push up with the pelvis. The body should be in an arched position with the head slightly back.

➥ Hold for a count of ten.

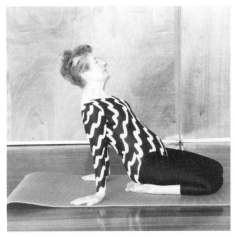

➤ Slowly lower yourself back onto your heels and curl forward to bring the head onto the floor in front of the knees. The arms should be in a relaxed position lying on the floor beside the lower legs, with the hands, palm-up, beside the feet. This is the pose of a child position from exercise fifteen and serves to redress the balance between the muscles on the front and the back of the body following the back-arched position.

➤ Slowly bring yourself to an upright position.

➤ Take five deep breaths before proceeding to the next exercise.

Question

Should I find the pelvic stretch demanding?

Answer

Yes, but as long as you do not find problems with your knees it is worth including, because it benefits so much of the body and is one of the rejuvenators.

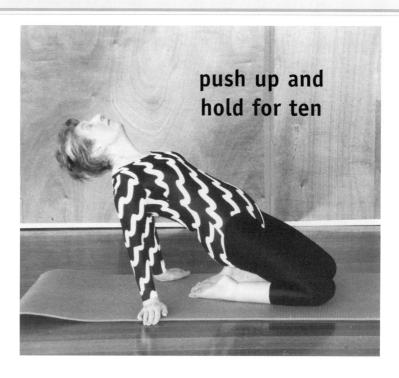

push up and
hold for ten

Exercise 18: Alternate leg raise

Benefit: Toning and firming for tired legs and feet, also acts on the hip flexors and to some extent on the abdominal muscles.

➤ Stretch out on the floor, lying on the back with the hands by the side of the body.

➤ Bend the right knee and place the foot flat on the floor beside the left knee.

➤ Point the toes of the left foot and raise the leg upwards towards the ceiling or as high as is comfortable for you.

➤ Keep the leg still and circle the foot slowly three times to the right and then three times to the left. You want the foot to travel through as large a circle as possible in order that the ankle mobility is maximised.

➤ Lower the leg gently to the floor and repeat on the other side.

➤ Repeat twice more on each side.

➤ Take three deep breaths before proceeding to the next exercise.

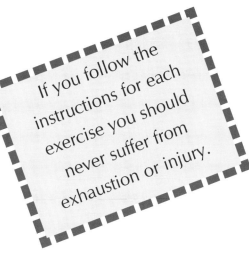

In the standing position the back of the knee should never be tight but soft.

If you follow the instructions for each exercise you should never suffer from exhaustion or injury.

Exercise 19: The clasp

Benefit: Excellent on shoulders and relieves tension. A must for good posture.

This exercise can be done standing or sitting.

Take the right stretched arm and hand over your right shoulder then let the elbow bend so that the hand drops down to touch the back.

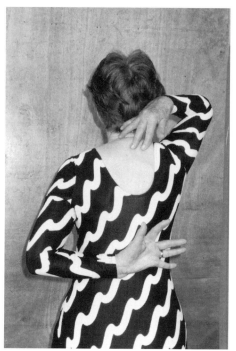

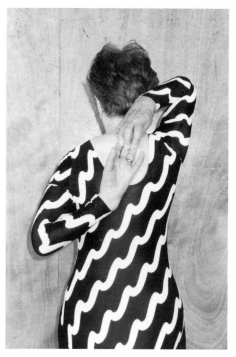

hold for ten

Work the hand as far down your back as you can.

Now take the left hand up behind your back and endeavour to link the fingers of your left hand with those of your right hand.

Hold for a count of ten.

If you have difficulty use a belt or rolled towel in the upper hand, grasp it with the other hand and gradually work at moving the hands closer together. This will take a number of sessions to achieve but you will soon find that you do not require the belt or towel.

Repeat the exercise with the left arm going over the shoulder and the right arm coming up from behind.

Breathe deeply five times before proceeding to the next exercise.

Question: Why am I nowhere near doing the clasp?

Answer: To begin with you are not alone with this difficulty. You obviously have stiff shoulder joints and tight shoulder muscles. If you have a belt in the arm that goes over the shoulder, you can grip the other end of it with the other hand and by working the hands along the belt fairly quickly you will manage to get the fingers to meet. Keep trying. It really loosens up the shoulder area and straightens the upper back. Remember to do the exercise with both the right and left arm at the top so that you develop the mobility in both shoulders.

you might need help to get started

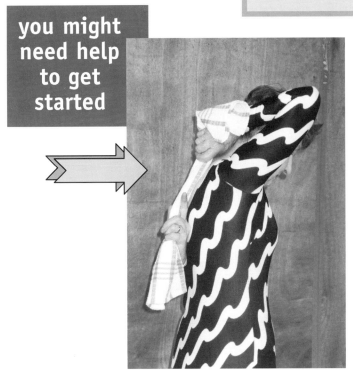

65

Exercise 20: Tranquil pose

Benefit: A truly restful pose once mastered. Good for the mobility of the spine.

Sit with the legs bent and the feet flat on the floor.

Lean forward prior to rocking backwards to move the weight from the hips up the spine and onto the shoulders.

As the weight rocks along the back towards the shoulders, the upper arms come onto the floor and the hands move in to support the lower back.

To facilitate the rolling-backwards movement it is important to maintain a rounded ball-like shape, i.e., a tucked position with the knees towards the chest and the head forwards.

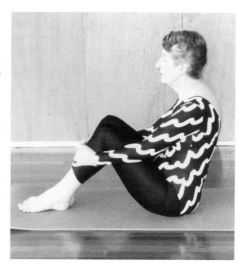

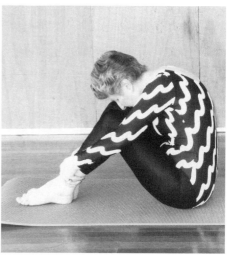

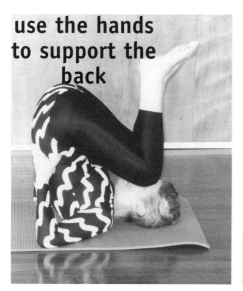

use the hands to support the back

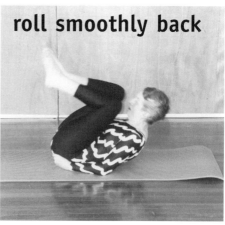

roll smoothly back

Once you feel in a stable and balanced position on the shoulders, straighten the legs. The legs should be pointing backwards over the head and approximately parallel to the floor. Probably for the first few sessions you will be content to do the exercise to this stage and develop your confidence in the rolling-back and balancing-on-the-shoulders stages.

straighten the legs

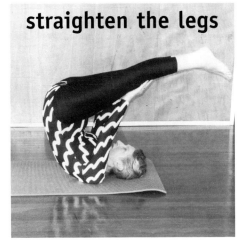

Transfer the hands from supporting the back to a position where the hands can support the knees of the outstretched legs.

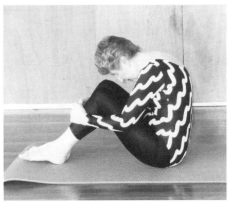

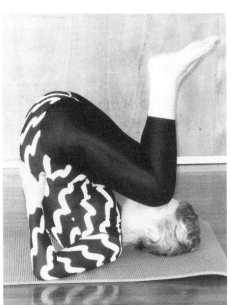

Hold for a count of ten. Gradually over time increase the count to twenty or thirty.

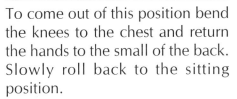

To come out of this position bend the knees to the chest and return the hands to the small of the back. Slowly roll back to the sitting position.

Breathe deeply five times before progressing to the next exercise.

Question: Why do I come down with a bang to the floor in the tranquil pose?

Answer: You may have difficulty in controlling your descent. The rolling up and rolling down actions were specifically designed to cater for your age group. Therefore, remember to bring the knees in to the chest before rolling down. You should also return and practise more of the rock-'n'-roll exercise.

Exercise 21: Bent knee sit-up

Benefit: Toning of the abdominal muscles.

➤ Lie with the back on the floor with both knees bent and the feet close to the buttocks about hip-width apart.

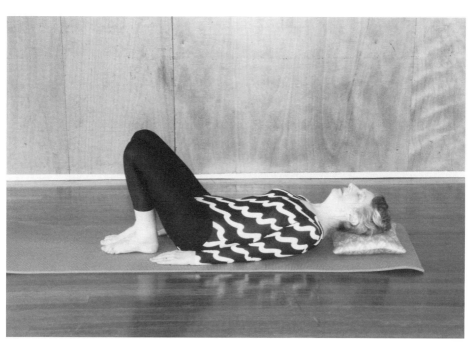

➤ Tilt the pelvis so that the small of the back (the flat area of the back just below the waist) is flat on the floor.

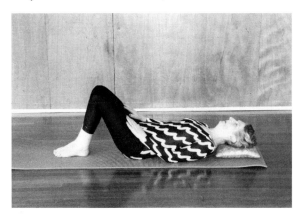

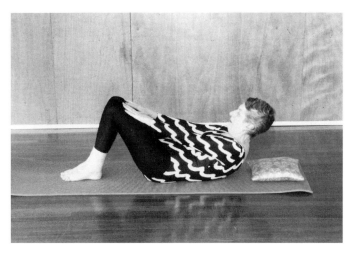

➤ Place the hands on the thighs and slowly raise the head and shoulders off the floor, sliding the hands along the thighs as you rise up. The head must be tilted forwards as you do this to avoid strain on the neck.

➤ Hold for a count of five and then slowly control the lowering of the back, shoulders and head to the floor.

➤ Repeat twice more. This can be increased to five then eight then ten repetitions over a period of weeks.

➤ Take five deep breaths before progressing to the next exercise.

Exercise 22: Knee and thigh stretch

Benefit: Tones the inner thighs.

➢   Sit on the floor with the legs outstretched and the back straight.

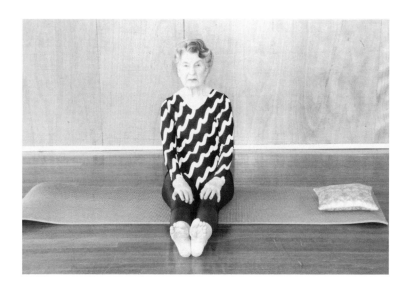

➢   Bend the knees outward and bring the soles of the feet together.

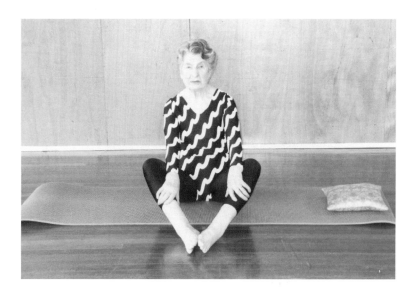

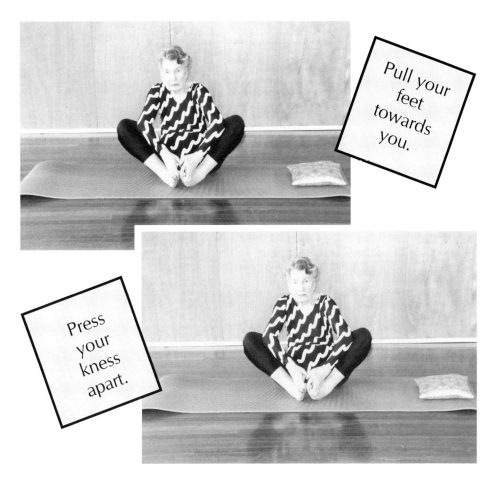

Pull your feet towards you.

Press your kness apart.

➢ Clasp the toes firmly with both hands and gently pull the feet as close to the body as is possible.

➢ Now try to take the thighs wider apart and lower the knees towards the floor. This can be aided by pulling the feet further towards you and also by gently pressing outward/downward on the thighs with the forearms. This pressure must be gentle and within the range of what is comfortable for you. Progress may be slow as this is quite a demanding exercise, but do not be tempted to rush things.

➢ Slowly release the position.

➢ Repeat three times.

➢ Take five deep breaths before progressing to the next exercise.

Exercise 23: Alternate nostril breathing

Benefit: Good for calming the mind. Relieves headaches and helps insomnia. Relieves tension. For maximum benefit it is wise to clear your nasal passages by blowing the nose before commencing this exercise.

➜ Sit on the floor in a way that is comfortable to you.

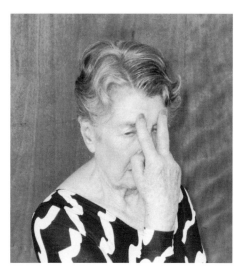

➜ Place your forefinger and middle finger of your right hand on your forehead, then close your right nostril with the thumb of the same hand.

➜ Breathe deeply through the left nostril, then close it with the ring finger.

➜ Count four then release the thumb and breathe out through the right nostril.

➜ Breathe in through the right nostril, close it with the thumb, count four then remove the ring finger and breathe out through the left nostril.

➜ Ideally the rhythm of breathing should be: breathe in for a slow count of six, hold for a count of four, breathe out for a count of six, in a continuous rhythmic manner.

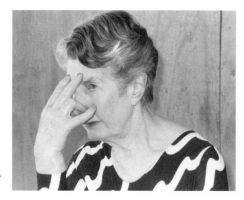

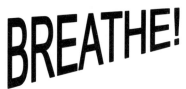

BREATHE!

Exercise 24: Roar

Benefit: Tones the facial and neck muscles. It is helpful to tone the neck muscles and relieves tension.

Sit comfortably on the floor with the legs crossed.

Purse the lips as if to whistle but breathe in.

Open the mouth really wide so that you stretch the entire face and stick the tongue out towards the chin as you breathe out to a count of five.

Repeat four more times.

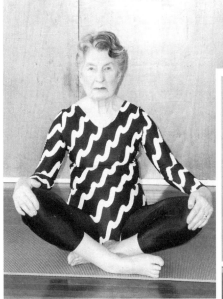

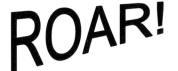

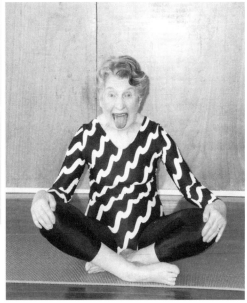

Exercise 25: Blindfold

Benefit: Excellent for tired eyes.

➤ Sit comfortably on the floor.

➤ Rub the palms and heels of the hand vigorously against each other until they feel hot, immediately cover the closed eyes with the cupped hands, one over each eye, for a count of twenty.

> **Writing up your notes
> each time you exercise
> shows your progress and
> becomes most interesting reading.**

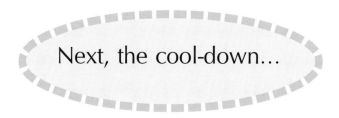

Next, the cool-down...

The cool-down

The cool-down is a relaxing but very important part of any programme of exercise. The aim is to return the body to the previous state with regard to temperature and heart rate. As it is not really very active it may seem unimportant, but it is in fact very important for your general well-being. It comprises one main exercise incorporating breathing and relaxation.

At the end of the cool-down there should be a marked feeling of relaxation. It should be difficult to raise either the arm or leg from the floor. Rectify this before rising by stretching and taking a few deep breaths.

It is very important to go through the cool-down as it restores the body and organs to a normal state.

The complete breathe

➤ Finish your programme by relaxing lying on your mat.

➤ Lie with the body on the back in a straight line, feet apart and turned outwards, hands by your side, palms upwards, fingers relaxed and slightly curled.

➤ Close the eyes to aid concentration.

➤ Start the deep breathing by raising the abdomen. This encourages the filling of the lower part of the lungs first. This should take three or five seconds. Now concentrate on expanding the rib cage to fill the upper part of the lungs. This should take a further three to five seconds. Inhalation should be through the nose.

➤ Exhale fully by pulling in the abdomen and emptying the lungs. Exhalation is through the mouth.

➤ Repeat four more times, finishing each outward breath with the lips parting and a final 'phoo' through parted lips, resulting in a complete relaxation.

➤ You should remain in this position for about five minutes to allow for recovery from exercise. Unless it is very warm you will probably want a sweater to prevent you from cooling down too much.

➤ Rise very slowly from this. Turn on to either side, draw the knees up towards the chest and clasp the hands under your chin. Rest in this position until you feel ready to rise.

Question Why do I sometimes not feel relaxed in the flat lying position?

Answer You may not be lying in a straight line with legs together, feet apart and turned out, which is the most natural relaxed position. Your shoulders should be down, well away from your ears. The body should be limp, not trying to hold a position.

Shortened programmes

In our busy lives we do not always have the time to do a full exercise programme likely to take up a complete hour. This section presents the programme in shorter groups of exercises that you can use on days when you want to exercise but are short of time. These shortened programmes are fairly well balanced in themselves, but you should do a different one each day and not pick the one you like and keep repeating it. The full programme covers the full range of exercises, taking all the main joints and their movements. The shorter variations, while balanced, cannot cover all joints/movements in the one programme. They do, however, still include the warm-up and cool-down as both are essential to safe exercise and should not be missed out.

Although these are shortened versions they are still well balanced in terms of the range of movements that they cover and they still require to be well executed. The aim is still to exercise and breathe deeply and thus improve posture, acquire greater ease of movement and a toning of the muscles. You will still benefit physically and mentally and as long as you persevere the results will please you. Whether it is the long or the short programme that you are doing, you start with a warm-up with the marching exercises and you finish with a cool-down to return the body to normal. Thus you will ensure that it is safe exercising.

The following three programmes present shortened versions that are still balanced but that should be done in rotation so that all exercises are done in the week.

PROGRAMME 1

Warm-up

Exercise 9(a) and (b), stepping
Exercise 2, shoulder shrug
Exercise 5, left and right side stretch
Exercise 12, hamstring and calf stretch
Exercise 6, sit on hands
Exercise 3, stretch

Main exercises

Exercise 1, long stretch and sit up
Exercise 6, rock-'n'-roll
Exercise 7, back massage and side rock
Exercise 9, cross legged elbow to knee rotations
Exercise 8, forehead to knee
Exercise 17, pelvic stretch
Exercise 15, pose of a child
Exercise 13, the cat
Exercise 14, cat stretch
Exercise 11, twist sitting up
Exercise 2, forward bend sitting
Exercise 4, alternate leg stretch
Exercise 19, the clasp
Exercise 24, roar
Cool-down

PROGRAMME 2

Warm-up

Exercise 9(c) and (d), stepping
Exercise 4(a) and (b), chin stretch and neck rolls
Exercise 6, sit on hands
Exercise 11, tree
Exercise 8, pendulum
Exercise 3, stretch

Main exercises

Exercise 1, long stretch and sit up
Exercise 6, rock-'n'-roll
Exercise 5, hip rotation
Exercise 21, bent knee sit up
Exercise 22, knee and thigh stretch
Exercise 15, pose of a child
Exercise 13, the cat
Exercise 14, cat stretch
Exercise 10, twist lying down
Exercise 12, cobra
Exercise 2, forward bend sitting
Exercise 4, alternate leg stretch
Exercise 18, alternate leg raise
Exercise 23, alternate nostril breathing
Exercise 20, tranquil pose
Cool-down

PROGRAMME 3

Warm-up

Exercise 9(e) and (f), stepping
Exercise 4, chin stretch and neck rolls
Exercise 7, twist
Exercise 6, sit on hands
Exercise 10, press-up standing
Exercise 3, stretch

Main programme

Exercise 1, long stretch and sit up
Exercise 6, rock-'n'-roll
Exercise 7, back massage and side rock
Exercise 8, forehead to knee
Exercise 16, head to floor
Exercise 3, breathing through nose
Exercise 13, the cat
Exercise 14, cat stretch
Exercise 15, pose of a child
Exercise 12, the cobra
Exercise 11, twist sitting up
Exercise 2, forward bend sitting
Exercise 4, alternate leg stretch
Exercise 25, blindfold
Exercise 20, tranquil pose
Cool-down

Other aspects of your overall fitness

By now you will have realised that the main emphasis of this programme is on stretching, muscle toning and breathing. These very essential elements of exercise however miss out one vital area of overall fitness, important for you if you want to be at your best and able to operate to your maximum. This is the area of cardio-vascular or cardio-respiratory fitness, and is concerned with the ability of your heart to deal with supplying adequate oxygen for the needs of the body. A strong heart and lungs will function most effectively and be able to supply the required quantities of oxygen carrying blood round the body, to meet the physical demands in a range of normal and mildly strenuous everyday situations.

Most people who have not pursued exercise seriously throughout their life do not relish the prospect of extensive vigorous exercise of an exhausting nature, in the forms of aerobics classes, circuit training or distance running, etc. It is also true that as we reach our later years our bodies are not well structured to withstand the pressures and impact of road running or all the stepping involved in step and aerobics classes, unless they are particularly carefully arranged to be low-impact and specifically for the older age group.

It is therefore important to look at the other aspects of your lifestyle, to see what you could incorporate into it to promote cardio-respiratory fitness. There are a number of things that you almost certainly do some of already, which you could adapt slightly. I am going to focus on developing this area rather than looking at persuading you to take up circuit training or some other very energetic sports activity.

For example you might:

do gardening
do the housework
go for the papers or odd bits of shopping locally
take the dog out/go for walks
play with grandchildren
go swimming
ride a bike
play golf
do other sports, e.g. skiing

If you do any of these things, and I am sure that all of us do several of them, you can think about how you do them and devise a strategy to adapt them slightly. In that way they will serve both their original functional purpose and also as an element of your health and exercise programme, without adding yet something else for you to fit into your busy life. I will take each of these possibilities in turn and suggest an approach that would help to make the activity serve the double purpose. Firstly I will explain briefly and simply what you should be doing in order to improve the functioning of your heart and lungs.

Our increasingly sedentary lifestyle, both at work and in our leisure, together with our increasing reliance on the car as a means of transport, creates problems for our heart and lungs. If we do not use them fully they become weaker and less efficient in their function. There are many aspects to endurance. For most of us the important area, where we need to do some work to improve our condition to meet the demands of an active everyday life, is to do with that type of endurance that is known as aerobic endurance. It is the normal supply of oxygen to the body that keeps us going throughout our daily activities and copes with the slight increases in effort from time to time. It is the capacity that enables us to go for a brisk walk, swim a few lengths of the pool, carry our suitcase up the stair or the railway platform, or put on that little spurt to get to the bus without gasping and wheezing. In other words, those everyday activities that put us under that little bit more stress than normal. These are the activities where the muscle-work involved requires an increase in the amount of oxygen supplied by the heart and lungs. If our heart and lungs have not been trained to meet these slight increases in demand then there is a shortage of oxygen and we gasp and puff laboriously to try to overcome it. In order to improve the condition of the heart and lungs it has been shown that we need to put ourselves under conditions that demand extra oxygen for a period of *at least twenty minutes about three times a week*. This can be done in a variety of ways, involving any of the activities listed above or many others. For many people, who are not seriously into sport and exercise, this is often most easily achieved by walking. If you have a dog or if you live somewhere that you can get a twenty-minute walk going to collect the newspapers, that is ideal. If you are accustomed to go swimming but normally just swim a little and float around and talk to friends for the rest of the time then you might need to think about restructuring the time that you spend at the pool to give you a spell of twenty minutes work at your fitness. You will obviously be wondering how hard you are supposed to work during this time. There are several ways of judging this. You can either take your heart rate, which will give you a reasonably accurate measure of how hard you are working, compared with how hard you require to work. Alternatively, if you are not into such specific methods of monitoring, you can work on the basis of assessing how hard you are working yourself. You are working sufficiently hard if you can *just manage to keep up a conversation with someone while you do the exercise*. If you are walking so fast that you are so out of breath that you cannot keep the conversation going, then you are working too hard for your current state of fitness. You need to slow down a little until you can just manage to talk while walking. If you are not feeling even slightly under pressure in relation to your breathing, then you need to increase the pace a bit.

If you want to measure your heart rate occasionally to see how you are getting on or to check that your idea of keeping talking/just slightly out of breath is correct, then these are the guidelines that you should follow. Walk for about five minutes briskly at what you think is the correct pace and then stop to take your pulse. You will need to be wearing a watch with a second hand as you are going to count the number of heart beats in six seconds. Take your pulse either on your wrist or preferably on your neck. If taking the pulse on the neck find your windpipe (which runs straight down the front of the neck), feel round the side of it between it and the muscle that runs down the side of the neck about an inch/two inches below the jaw bone. You should find the pulse quite easy to locate when you have been exercising.

What should your pulse be?

Your pulse, which is a reflection of your heart rate, depends on your age, your level of fitness and the level of activity when you take it. The following example shows you how to work out your personal target heart rate and gives you the target heart rate for people of fifty, sixty, and seventy years as a guide. Your personal target heart rate gives you a guide about the level of intensity of exercise that you should be working at to improve your fitness. It is based on a percentage of your maximum heart rate. When you first start an exercise programme you should start at a target of sixty per cent of maximum and as your fitness improves you should progress to seventy per cent of maximum, then seventy-five. Even for those that are very fit and motivated eighty per cent should be the maximum that they use as a target.

The following is an example for a person aged fifty

Subtract your age from 220, e.g. 220 (maximum heart rate in youth) minus 50 years equals 170.

Work out sixty per cent of that figure, e.g. sixty per cent of 170 equals 102. Also work out eighty per cent of that figure, e.g. eighty per cent of 170 equals 136.

A hundred and two beats per minute is the rate that you should be working at in order to make sixty per cent effort, and 136 beats per minute to work at eighty per cent effort. If you are currently quite unfit you should start at a target of sixty per cent (this may feel fairly tiring if you are starting off really unfit, but you will fairly quickly make progress), and gradually over a period of about three to four months work up to a target of seventy per cent, seventy-five per cent and even eighty per cent effort. As you become fitter you will need to challenge yourself more to achieve benefits. Never go above eighty per cent effort to improve your general fitness. Working harder than that will mean that you are improving other aspects that really are of little relevance to the more elderly participant who is involved for reasons of their general well-being and fitness for everyday life.

When you count your heart rate for six seconds (i.e. for one tenth of a minute) you should get a count of 10 (10 times 10 equals 100 beats per minute, which is near enough to 102 and is as accurate as you can get with this quick method of counting), for eighty per cent you'd get a count of 13 or 14 beats, which corresponds to a heart rate of 130 or 140 beats.

Fifty-year-olds

If you are approximately fifty years old the rate you want to exercise at to improve your endurance is 102 beats per minute (10 beats when you count for 6 seconds) to start with. This should go up to a maximum of 136 beats per minute (13 or 14 beats when you count for 6 seconds) when you are really fit.

Sixty-year-olds

If you are approximately sixty years old the rate you want to exercise at to improve your endurance is 96 beats per minute (9 or 10 beats when you count for 6 seconds) to start with. This should go up to a maximum of 128 beats per minute (12 beats when you count for 6 seconds) when you are really fit.

Seventy-year-olds

If you are approximately seventy years old the rate you want to exercise at to improve your endurance is 90 beats per minute (9 beats when you count for 6 seconds) to start with. This should go up to 120 beats per minute (12 beats when you count for 6 seconds) when you are really fit.

Remember that if you have any questions about your health or whether you should be undertaking an exercise programme you must consult you doctor before commencing this or any other exercise regime.

Try to manage to check your heart rate *occasionally* to confirm that you are working at a pace that really will do you some good. It is such a pity to do lots of potentially good work at just the wrong pace and thus not get the benefit. That is what happens if you work either too gently or indeed if you work too hard. Working too hard does not mean more improvement. Training of any type is specific, and that means that there is a specific level of effort that will help, and beyond that achieves no more. It just makes you tired and sore and generally wears you out unnecessarily.

Do not however become obsessed about it. For most people just 'feeling' how hard they are working will suffice. You should manage to do most exercise of this nature just using the idea of working hard enough so that you can *only just* maintain an intelligible conversation. Endeavour to apply these principles to any of the following activities, or others, that you do.

Gardening

If you have a garden and do all or most of the work in it yourself you will not only be getting quite a lot of exercise but also lots of fresh air, which is important in feeling that you are in good health. Most of us feel much better during the summer weather when there are many more hours of daylight, when the light is much brighter, when we get some sunshine and when we are able to get out and about more with a lot less clothing on to keep us warm. Use this gardening opportunity to the maximum. See it as an opportunity rather than a chore. Do the grass-cutting, light digging or hoeing and hedge-clipping at a brisk pace, remembering as you do so the good that it is doing you as well as the garden. Although gardening gives you lots of exercise in the form of bending and stretching, it is not necessarily the best cardio-respiratory exercise as you are not often involved in exercise of a continuous nature for any length of time. It will however undoubtedly help with your overall fitness. You can try to structure what you do to get aerobic benefit from it. For example you could perhaps do all the energetic tasks in the same gardening session of the week to try to get the maximum endurance benefit out of the activity. You can of course always apply the procedure of checking your heart rate to see if you are working hard enough to get endurance benefit.

Housework

Housework is something that most of us have to do a bit of. Again this can be another opportunity for exercise that will be of benefit rather than a chore to be done. Utilise all the necessary bending and stretching to give you some really good exercise. Hoover, dust and mop energetically. Do not avoid going up and down the stairs. That is one way of ensuring that activity around the house can be beneficial. Remember that you are trying to get a period of exercise that lasts about twenty minutes to be effective in improving the functioning of your heart and lungs. Again remember to check up on your rate of work to see if it really is helping you. It is amazing how much mopping, vacuuming and polishing you can get done in twenty minutes at the right pace!

Walking

This can be to get the papers or small bits of shopping or taking the dog out. It is an ideal opportunity and one that is easy to adapt to ensure that the duration is twenty minutes and that the effort level is correct. If you live too close to the shops for the journey to take twenty minutes then you can extend it by going round another block or combine it with some other small local visit to be done. Come and go by the long route to the shops. Whatever you do, do not take the car. Remember to walk briskly, breathe deeply and check your pace to ensure that it will serve the two functions of getting the shopping and also of improving your aerobic fitness.

If you have a dog you have the ideal opportunity for lots of walking and you will have a very contented pet into the bargain. If you are in this fortunate position you should have no problems, as taking the dog out for two twenty-minute walks a day will ensure that your general fitness is very good as long as you remember to make sure that you are walking fast enough for it to be effective. Many such walks lose their fitness benefit when you meet a friend and stand and talk. Encourage them to go along with you on the walk rather than stand talking. You can always blame the dog saying that it gets impatient if you stop for long. You can then use talking to them as you walk to measure the intensity of your walking.

If you live in an area with nice country or parkland walks you are lucky and can easily make this a part of your lifestyle, knowing that it will be doing you lots of good physically as well as giving you the opportunity to enjoy the local countryside, see how the spring growth is coming on, etc. If you live in a town or city it is not as obvious but you can usually find somewhere that is both safe and interesting to walk, if you really think about it. It can sometimes be achieved by simply walking when you would normally have gone by car or bus. For example, walk to a friend's house, walk to the shops or walk to post a letter. Opportunities to walk can be found if you try. Our lack of walking is just that we have become too lazy and now think that even short distances are too far.

Cycling

If you have a bike, use it rather than the car. Use it to go for the papers or bits of shopping or simply go for a cycle ride to get some fresh air and exercise. Like walking it is always more pleasant if you live in an area with interesting scenery and quiet roads, but that is not essential. Cycling is also good as you are not weight-bearing on the legs, so it does not stress the hip and knee joints with impact pressure.

Grandchildren

Grandchildren can be a wonderful source of exercise. They also really appreciate the time that you can give them. Very often as their parents are busy working and running homes etc., no one else has time to play with them. Structure games activities around their interests, ensuring that the activity gives you some exercise of a fairly continuous nature. Take them swimming, take them to the park and play ball with them, or take the baby in the pram for a brisk walk.

Swimming

If you normally go swimming that is an ideal activity to review as a means of real endurance improvement. Swimming is the best activity for all forms of physical improvement as it is non-weight bearing and therefore does not put stress on the joints, and it also uses all the muscles of the body and can make as severe demands on the endurance of the body as you want. Swimming a number of lengths to take about twenty minutes and then floating and having a relaxing chat with friends can be achieved in about forty minutes. If you have not been swimming for many years except when you are on holiday give it some thought.

There are many really nice swimming pools now with lots of extra interesting features. They are probably much nicer than when you last went to the local baths. To start with set yourself a target of a number of lengths (possibly twelve to start with or twenty if you remember being a good swimmer) and see how long it takes you. You can then gradually increase the number of lengths and increase the pace of the swimming until you are sure that it is at the required level of effort to be of real benefit to your endurance capacity.

Golf

If you are a golfer you probably already do a lot of walking and get a certain amount and range of exercise from that. Due to the nature of the game and the social conventions associated with it, it is however most likely carried out too slowly and with too many pauses of some length to be of benefit to your endurance capacity. You need therefore to rethink your strategy if you are going to count this towards improving your endurance. This might include very brisk walking between shots. It might work in certain situations but in many cases you do not have sufficient control over the pace of the game. Maybe this is just an activity you enjoy and you are doing it purely for that. You are still getting significant exercise and lots of fresh air from it. It is just important that you do not think that it is giving you benefits that it is not.

Other sports

Perhaps you already participate in other sports activities. Assess that activity and work out if it is really helping your fitness. If it is not helping your fitness then continue doing it simply because you enjoy it, you get the fresh air and it has a good social side associated with it etc., and find something else to do to help your aerobic fitness.

For example, bowling will do little for your aerobic fitness whereas cross-country skiing will really help it. Playing cricket will do little for your fitness with all its standing around and intermittent activity, whereas cycling can be structured to help it a lot. The continuous nature of the activity, with few pauses, is important together with the fact that you can adjust the pace for yourself and maintain it for about twenty minutes.

General

You do not need to do the same activity three times a week or the same activity every week. There are many other activities that you may do that I have not covered. The important thing is to appreciate this area of need that you have in your exercise programme for all-round fitness and well-being. You need to look at the range of things that you do and see if there are three episodes per week of such activity that will genuinely stimulate your heart and breathing rate as has been suggested. If there are not then you need to look to see what you could do to improve the situation. Trying to use activities that you already do is a way of making them dual-purpose and still leaving you plenty of time to do all those other things that you want to do in your later years.

Conclusion

I have endeavoured to give you as much information as possible to enable you to carry out all the exercises without the presence of a teacher. You may think that there is a lot of reading to do before you really get going with the exercise. Yes, that is the case if you are going to know enough to work at the programme over a period of time, so that it will do you good and you will enjoy it. You do need to have an understanding of what you are doing.

Once you feel that you are making progress you will understand better why there is a greater emphasis on breathing and on shaking out the arms and legs regularly. The photographs will help you have a picture of what you are trying to do just as you would have a teacher to copy in a class. The benefits and the questions and answers I hope will clarify some of the things that you might have wanted to ask a teacher.

All aspects have been covered to enable you to exercise without injury or exhaustion. You will discover that the cool-down is just as important as the warm-up. Do try to write up your own notes of progress in the pages provided. This is particularly important initially and will give you the opportunity to identify your strengths and weaknesses and see a record of your progress. Your record of progress should really encourage you to keep going.

You will have days that do not please you and you will gradually come to realise the harmony within that exercise and breathing combined can bring you. You may well think that I have exaggerated when I said that you could feel ten years younger. I assure you that I meant exactly what I said. Why do you think I still exercise at eighty-seven years of age! I also told you that you would improve mentally and physically, and I really mean that. Remember that I started to exercise only at sixty years of age, and though my progress was variable I was still pleased with the results – so pleased that I just never think of giving up, even now. I recently had an accident and had a double fracture of my pelvis. I have been assured, by the hospital and the various doctors, nurses and physiotherapists that looked after me during my recovery, that I was out of hospital and at home living alone again within eleven days due to the fact that I was fit and motivated. I am also assured that my recovery has been as good as it has been due to my previous exercise experience, general muscle condition and my motivation to get back to exercising again.

I cannot finish without touching on diet or eating habits, as I do not believe in fashionable diets. If you enjoy the programme and can see the results I feel that you will also adjust your eating habits if you need to. I sometimes put on a few pounds and tackle it by eating roughly half of what I normally eat. I also cut down generally on fats and sugars until the excess weight has gone. This is where mental strength comes in, because it is easier to discipline yourself.

I wish you happy, enjoyable and beneficial exercising and very long, active and enjoyable later years.

PERSONAL EXERCISE RECORD

PERSONAL EXERCISE RECORD

PERSONAL EXERCISE RECORD

PERSONAL EXERCISE RECORD

PERSONAL EXERCISE RECORD

PERSONAL EXERCISE RECORD

PERSONAL EXERCISE RECORD

PERSONAL EXERCISE RECORD